COMMON SENSE NUTRITION

A Pragmatic Approach to an Issue Made Complicated

Colin E. Champ, M.D., C.S.C.S.

CDR Health & Nutrition Publishing
Pittsburgh, PA

"The simple things are also the extraordinary things, and only the wise can see them."

- Paulo Coelho

"Any intelligent fool can make things bigger, more complex, and more violent. It takes a touch of genius—and a lot of courage—to move in the opposite direction."

- Albert Einstein

"Tell me what you eat and I will tell you who you are."

- Jean Anthelme Brillat-Savarin

For Juli, Aurelia, and Chiara

Contents

PROLOGUE

The following book was written based upon thousands of interactions with clients and friends during my nutrition and exercise sessions with them. In the early stages of my medical career, this would often occur via one-on-one conversations. However, once I realized that the vast majority of individuals seeking guidance on nutrition and exercise were having the same concerns and confusion about food and thus asking the same questions over and over again, I realized I could be more efficient in my outreach and dissemination of information by conducting group sessions. Thus, was born Dr. Champ's "Nutrition Sessions" at the Exercise Oncology and Resiliency Center (EOC) that I established and operate in Pittsburgh, Pennsylvania. The EOC is located in Bellevue, an area smack dab in the center of Greater Pittsburgh. This steel town suburb was named by its initial Italian inhabitants and apparently had a pretty nice view (bella view = Bellevue). Like many areas of Pittsburgh, when the steel mills closed in the '70s and '80s, the local economy contracted, leaving many of Bellevue's residents near or below the poverty line.

However, like most Pittsburghers, Bellevue is composed of gritty and resilient fighters, leaving these sessions as incredibly honest discussions about all aspects of food imaginable.

These sessions have gradually morphed into "ask me anything" sessions where we take deep dives into the ins and outs of nutrition, cancer, and what it takes to maintain a healthy lifestyle. While sitting on the turf floor in the back corner of the facility (affectionately named "The Pit") casually discussing food and nutrition, the discussion would inevitably turn to the roots of some of the more common modern food recommendations or demonizations, then mushroom into broader conversations. What I have come to realize over the years is that while these sessions are open discussions designed for me to answer questions with my own expertise, oftentimes I learn more than the participants, ever-sharpening my razor to cut through the polarity, nuances, and misinformation circulating throughout society. I've learned what the media—unfortunately the most common source of misinformation—is telling us to eat or do, as well as new and updated misconceptions about food. I've learned about the infatuation modern society has with technology and how it is using it to complicate what were once straightforward aspects of daily life. And I've learned about the tendency toward choosing comfort and ease over health when approaching food, the massively negative impact of consumerism on health and eating, the disconnect with food and cooking, and the inconsistencies in human habits when it comes to approaching food.

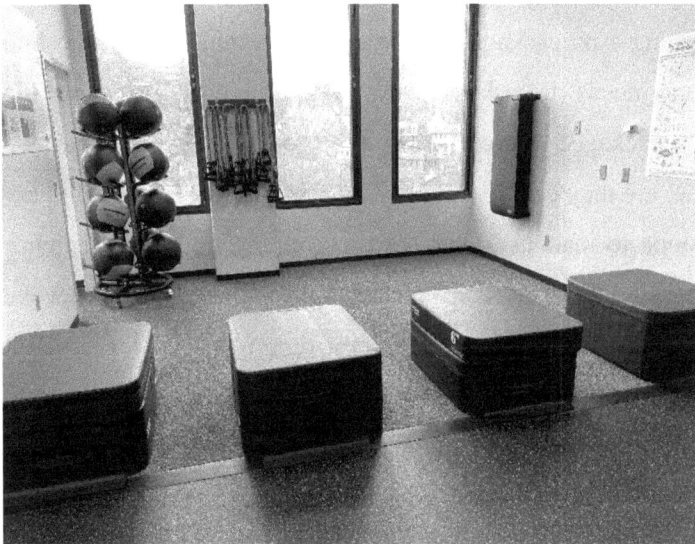

We hold these sessions at the EOC face-to-face, with no remote video allowed. Having a real, open, authentic and intimate conversation that is sensitive and nonjudgmental is absolutely required in this setting. Academic theories do not work here; this is real life and people want answers, solutions and takeaways they can put directly into practice. These individuals earnestly want to improve their lives, and for many of them, past advice and societal pressures just aren't working to put them in a healthy place. While these conversations often end with "Can't you just tell us what to eat?", the importance of not taking a shortcut and talking through their relationship with food and those around them is vital. For instance, if someone is derailing their entire day by eating a prepackaged breakfast on the run, the key question one needs to ask is why this individual is eating the prepackaged food and why on the go. Do they like the taste—i.e. are they eating primarily for pleasure, which is a slippery slope to maneuver—or are they relying on its convenience because they stayed up late last night on their device and woke up late, and thus it is actually a time management issue? It might even be that, with all the buzzword-of-the-moment "healthy" ingredients slapped across the appealingly-designed packaging, they think that this particular processed food is "good for you" and thus good for them. Simply telling someone what to eat or avoid is like reading an Italian dictionary and then being surprised when you aren't actually able to speak Italian.

What factors lead you or me to eat a certain food is likely well beyond the food itself. And the physical and physiologic result of eating a certain food is definitely well beyond the food itself. In other words, foods and the ways in which we have obtained the foods send our body a message. By consuming "instant" meals and prepackaged processed foods, we are telling ourselves that food is a readily available convenience item and thus we do not have to work for it—going against how our bodies and minds approached food for almost the entirety of human history. This can have implications beyond the immediate sugar rush—and inevitable subsequent crash—from a nutrient-sparse, readily available pastry in the morning, or alternatively how a nutrient-dense breakfast might signal to your body and brain that it's "go time" and you're priming yourself for a successful day. Did you go to bed earlier to get up earlier to make breakfast after a full eight hours of sleep? Or is your morning a haphazard and chaotic sprint from the second the alarm clock goes off? More to come later on both of these scenarios. (An important introductory note: if you consume foods that have adequate vitamins, minerals and nutrients and your body composition is optimal, then this book may be of less relevance to your situation, although it will serve as a handy refresher and motivating reinforcement to keep doing what you're doing.)

While the continuing in-person discussions with clients in "The Pit" are and will always remain invaluable, I eventually caved to unrelenting demand and decided to write this brief book telling people what to eat. However, I've expanded my original blueprint of my noble mission to include HOW to eat. This book is a quick, handy reference and certainly does not contain all of the required knowledge on the subject, but it hits the high points that are frequently recurring in my discussions with clients. Finding, cooking, preparing and eating food is a vital part of every human life and constitutes a lifelong journey, one whose path is not decided upon after reading a single book. Like everything worthwhile in this life of ours, following a healthy path takes dedication and effort, as does getting back on track whenever we happen to fall off. Though in reality, what to eat and how to eat is less complicated than people usually think, and these not-so-secret secrets have been disclosed time and again over the past thousand years, for our industrially-starved ancestors had no choice but to push for nutritious natural foods and prepare them as such. It is humorous to me to witness academics in their ivory towers skew or altogether botch nutrition and healthy lifestyle tenets repeatedly, while Italian immigrants from Calabria working in steel mills in Pittsburgh with no educational background knew how to get it right a century ago.

Enjoy this quick read. And if you want to learn more after doing so, head out to Pittsburgh for a few lively

"Nutrition Sessions" with us at the Exercise Oncology & Resiliency Center.

Colin E. Champ, MD, CSCS

September, 2024

1

THE FIVE RULES OF EATING

L et's face it: we all love to make out the act of eating to be more complicated than it is. In particular, food companies often complicate and obfuscate the food equation and then proceed to provide solutions to this complex problem that seemingly always involves consumers buying more of their products. An infamous example of such "solutions" was SnackWell's cookies, which apparently solved the "new" problem of avoiding fat after the Food Pyramid and low-fat craze swept through the US in the '80s and '90s. Thankfully SnackWell's is now out of business; similarly, several "fake" meat companies are no longer fooling the public and will likely be shuttering their doors soon. (Yes, I said "fake" as opposed to "impossible" or any of this product's other masqueraded adjectives which imply "not real" in a more alluring manner.)

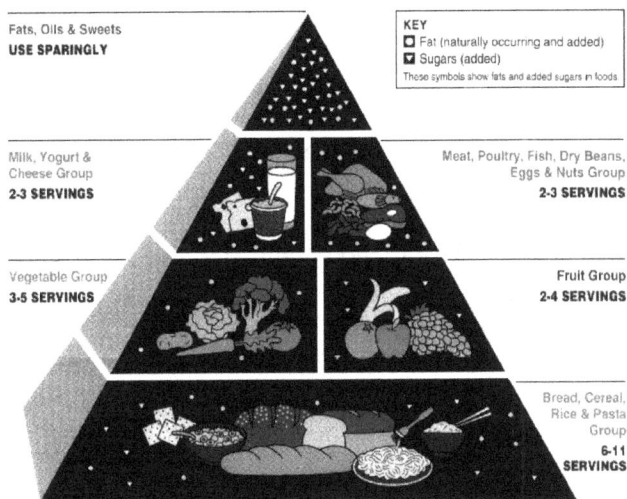

Fats, Oils & Sweets
USE SPARINGLY

KEY
☐ Fat (naturally occurring and added)
☑ Sugars (added)
These symbols show fats and added sugars in foods

Milk, Yogurt &
Cheese Group
2-3 SERVINGS

Meat, Poultry, Fish, Dry Beans,
Eggs & Nuts Group
2-3 SERVINGS

Vegetable Group
3-5 SERVINGS

Fruit Group
2-4 SERVINGS

Bread, Cereal,
Rice & Pasta
Group
**6-11
SERVINGS**

The original Food Pyramid recommended a gut-exploding 11 servings of bread, rice, and pasta per day, ushering in 50 plus years of societal carb-loading.

These "solutions" purport to solve a problem that did not exist in the first place, and more often than not they make the problem worse. The anti-fat craze was followed by decades of skyrocketing obesity. Call it a coincidence (I don't), but the drastic change in the human body habitus during this time is unparalleled compared to any other point in the entire history of our species: we once grew erect and upright, we now grow horizontal. The producers of the "healthy" fake meat Soylent Green products told us they were going to save the environment. Ponder that one: mashing together a hodgepodge of upwards of 30 chemicals into a pink goo and shipping it all over the world is going to save both our health and the environment. History and half a brain strongly suggest the only people this was benefiting were the shareholders of the pink goo companies and their pawns as they receive their payouts, yet we are supposed to believe the companies (and academic overlords) who tell us this is how we should eat.

When it comes to food, we are bombarded with advertisements to no end promising fake fixes to all our food and health woes. As an example of this insanity, I remember as a child watching my cartoons after a half day of kindergarten and being bombarded with commercial after commercial of "Fruit" by the Foot, Teddy Grahams, "Fruit" Roll Ups, Little Debbies and a barrage of nutrient-sparse snacks masquerading as food. Looking back, I am appalled at the pompous audacity of these brands to use the word "fruit" to describe themselves, and to make matters worse many had "heart healthy" labels on them too! Wash them down with Kool-Aid or Capri Sun and you've got yourself a sugar bomb with no nutrition whatsoever—the last thing we should be advertising to children who need huge amounts of vitamins and nutrients to grow and properly develop both body and mind. Sugar is an addictive drug, and these snack companies intend to get users craving that sweet taste early on in life.

Nature never planned for us to go from breast milk, one of the most nutrient-dense foods available, to sugar bomb "fruit" snacks. And on top of that, being inundated with these prepackaged processed snacks teaches us at a young age that food is always instantly available. Even a nursing baby must work for its sustenance. Nature, however, does not have shareholders or board members clamoring for her to produce revenue. With the natural order of things upended, unnatural monsters like cavities and obesity would soon follow.

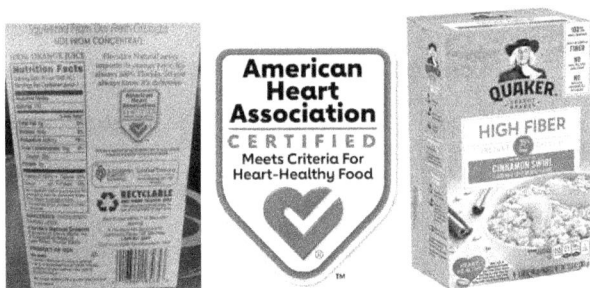

"Heart Healthy" labels can be found scattered across numerous children's cereals, as well as orange juice and other high-carbohydrate foods. One serving of instant oatmeal contains 34g of carbs, only 4g of protein and 12% of the daily allowance of added sugar. Add some skim milk and wash it down with some heart healthy orange juice, and you may reach 100 grams of sugar by breakfast. Perhaps it is time to start labeling foods as "muscle-healthy" and "brain-healthy."

Yet these foods illustrate the food mindset well, and for most of society this mindset continues from childhood through adolescence and well into adulthood. Perhaps we simply never want to grow up, but the number of adults who continue to rely on their prepackaged "fruit" snacks and pretend they are healthy is quite worrisome. It is hard, if not altogether impossible, to argue that this is a healthy or sustainable way to eat, yet many nutrition "authorities" and advertising companies never seem to stop pushing this message down our throats. The mania has recently reached its peak, with America's nutritional recommendation committees now prescribing various forms of a "healthy" processed food diet.[1] Again, we must ask ourselves: Who is this healthy for? We the People, or the corporations selling us processed junk and the shareholders whose pockets they line?

A common discussion topic at our Nutrition Sessions is to cut through this smoke-and-mirrors confusion and agenda-backed insanity—there are no special interest groups in The Pit, just a bunch of people that want to get back to being healthy. In fact, this is the easiest navigable area of food that thus allows us to cut to the chase.

We eat for five main reasons:

1.   To supply the vitamins and minerals required for our body and cells to function

2.   To acquire nutrient building blocks required for our body and cells to function (e.g. protein for muscle, fats for cell membranes and nerves, small amounts of carbohydrates for glycogen, etc.)

3.   To provide non-nutritive substances that stress our cells with "chemical" nutrients like polyphenols and phytochemicals and feed our bowel bacteria with fiber

4.   To provide fuel to burn (though most of us consume too much fuel)

5.   To provide emotional pleasure, via a) social connection with friends and family and b) introspective and meditative benefits of the process of food preparation

Notice that convenience is NOT one of the reasons why we eat. Many clients and friends have argued to add to the fifth item above the benefit of connecting spiritually with past cultures, ancestors and nature. I wholeheartedly agree with this and would not mind if you penciled it in as c) to bullet number 5. As for 5b), I have always held in high personal regard the almost magical ability of the food preparation process to channel innate mechanisms buried deep within us.

Hot take: have you ever noticed that those same influencer self-help gurus (the ones with all the pictures of themselves on their social media pages) will try to sell you premade packaged foods (of which they get a cut) and in the next breath tell you the importance of meditation (while having someone post pictures of them meditating)? The majority of these snake-oil salesmen (and saleswomen) have likely never prepared a meal, because if so, they wouldn't be so starved for quiet peace of mind. Meal preparation is one of man's oldest forms of meditation, and it confers the same mind-clearing benefits as humming and touching one's fingertips to each other while sitting in a cross-legged Zazen position. That being said, preparing meals is a tradeoff that requires putting in effort in exchange for taking out the middleman. If you are not paying anyone to prepare a meal for you, someone else's profit-making machine takes a hit while your mental health takes a boost. The point is that eating and preparing food are, and always have been, integral components of our daily lives, and up until relatively recently we never simply snapped our fingers—or pushed a button on an app—and had food waiting for us.

When considering the above list of reasons why we eat, the order of the listed items is also important. For instance, if you are turning to number 4 or 5 before 1-3, you may find yourself in trouble. If your first meal of the day could be described as carb-loading (i.e. fuel to burn) or if you are eating a meal merely because it tastes good yet violates 1-3, you may find yourself in trouble. This is the most common way in which individuals derail their nutrition. While eating primarily for pleasure can rob us of our required vitamins, minerals, building blocks and healthy cellular chemicals, eating primarily for pleasure is a slippery slope that gets a person perceiving food as a psychological tool as opposed to a vital fuel for life. For such individuals, food can more closely resemble an addictive drug as opposed to an essential lifeline. This reversal of roles can lead individuals on a path of addictive craving, binge eating and subsequent self-resentment. This perception of food was literally force-fed to me and many other children through the parade of Dunkaroos and Teddy Grahams TV commercials, embedding messages deep within our brains that such foods were normal. And I had the cavities to prove it. (In his must-read book Amusing

Ourselves to Death, Neil Postman points to television as the major issue in the equation; I urge you to pick that book up next once you finish with mine.).

A key takeaway from the above is that we eat food to obtain nutrition and not to avoid it. The food pyramid, calorie-counting methodologies, angry dietitians advising their clients to avoid this and that, all espouse a global reductionist strategy—advising us to eat to avoid. While we clearly need to avoid certain foods, particularly artificial and "fake" foods, our mindset must return to one of gathering (and hunting) food to acquire our bodies' required nutrition—not this constant over-emphasis on reduction. We eat food to obtain adequate vitamins, nutrients, minerals and essential materials to convert into the bricks and mortar of our bodies, period. For many of us, consuming food with the goal of achieving adequate protein will magically push our entire eating habits in the right direction. If we are eating to achieve adequate protein and vitamins, we will naturally avoid the Entenmann's cookies— they serve utterly no purpose in our pursuit to create necessary building blocks, but merely are a drug providing nothing more than short-lived pleasure. When we start avoiding the foods that make us feel terrible afterwards and do little to satiate our hunger, it gets easier to stay on track.

As a side note, if someone, like a dietitian or nutritionist, is telling you to follow an eating pattern that would be considered carb-loading, and you are not a lineman attempting to gain weight in the off season or training for the Olympics, run.

Taking a pure reductionist approach, you can eat those cookies but you must cut something else out to keep the overall negative intake amount low. You can then count calories and check off that box but will likely end up with inadequate nutrition for the day. According to this calorie-counting strategy, you must avoid higher fat foods even though they are often higher in protein and vitamins, all because they tip the calories ledger past the limit. It is like a game of golf—eating with the strategy of keeping your score low. But this approach is a surefire recipe for failure, supported by both analytical data and the anecdotal evidence observed in nature (and your grocery store). It is not a coincidence that most high-protein foods that are found abundantly in nature, and also on the perimeter of the grocery store, also contain a higher content of nutrients and vitamins, but also often contain some fat. The name fat-soluble vitamins says it all. These foods also happen to be satiating, solving the riddle of finding complete nutrition that also fills you up while ending the cycle that many of us have found ourselves stuck in throughout the past several decades. These are the kinds of foods that lead tortured souls to the Promised Land of healthy eating and disciplined dieting success.

2

MINIMIZING THE DETOURS: EATING FOR PLEASURE

I f you feel like the person I discussed in the last chapter may be you, a good exercise is to name the top five foods that make you lose control. What are those five foods that once you start eating, you lose all willpower and just cannot stop? Worse yet, what are those foods that make you crawl back to them shortly after regaining that willpower, sending you on a roller coaster of highs and lows?

Topping the list most often are cookies, cake, candy, chocolate, bread, bread with butter, potato chips, ice cream and pastries. There is a consistent theme with these foods: lots of sugar, grains and some fat, and maybe even some salt. Interestingly, if you remove the sugar and grains the binge eating tends to stop. Nobody loses control over eating pure butter, olive oil, or lard. Change high sugar milk chocolate to high fat and low sugar dark chocolate and few are taken on the one-way track to Bingetown. Bread is a common fuel for overeating, and while butter may accentuate the taste, the bread is the clear driver. Add some salt and you may have the trifecta, but remove the bread and the craving is curbed. There is a reason why many restaurants start the meal with a bread basket; they know that no matter how much you fill up on the bread, you will still be hungrier to purchase more of their food. There are several physiological mechanisms as to why this happens, but we will not dive into them here. You can check out my other books for a deeper dive.

Most of us have fallen into this trap. I have been part of endless bread baskets, and the name is not far from the truth. Worse yet, these "pleasure" foods result in a roller coaster physically and mentally when your blood sugar initially spikes, only to come crashing down. Your mood will follow the crash, leaving you sad and oftentimes craving more of the same food. That ice cream carton may end up empty in a couple hours, making these pleasure foods seem more like pain foods as you embark on a vicious cycle.

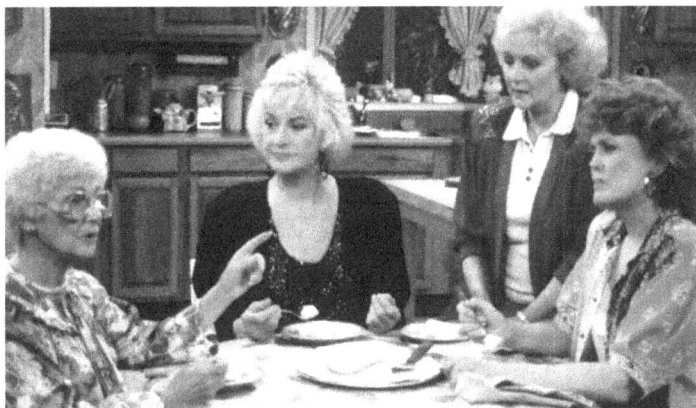

Sophia, Dorothy, Rose and Blanche enjoy a typical late-night cheesecake on *The Golden Girls*

But, but, but… you deserve it! I have heard this told to my cancer patients only a thousand or so times by their "friends" and even medical personnel, or perhaps worst of all their dietitians (see Chapter 5). Yet the reality is that this approach is akin to turning to food as a pleasure drug, and the side effects of the drug are severe. It may be a difficult discussion to tell someone undergoing treatment for a serious medical condition that perhaps that daily cookie is not the best idea, but we owe it to them to be 1000% honest, particularly when they are taking corticosteroids that already artificially increase their blood sugar levels. Anyone that tries to promote this drug-like behavior to you is not an ally, as anyone who has experienced this addictive behavior understands just how pathologic it can be. If you are able to eat those foods above in small amounts, close the lids and put them away for several weeks, I am impressed and sincerely congratulate you. However, if you are the remaining 99.9% of us, I would steer clear.

The latter point is an important one. The friends that surround you can serve to help you to make the right choices with food, or sit on your shoulder as the devil that goads you into eating those foods that derail all your efforts. Choose wisely, as the number of "friends" who will push to derail you, often to make themselves feel better, is unfortunately very high.

Avoiding the binge...

Have you ever been unable to stop eating steak, butter, bacon or another high protein, high fat food? Before you answer this, I dare you to give it a try. Go cook up a steak with a lot of salt or a dozen or more bacon strips, two foods that the calorie counters repeatedly tell you will kill you. What happens? Lo and behold, you quickly become full and don't want more. Try some other foods. Make a giant omelet with several whole eggs, some veggies, and raw cheese from grass-fed milk. You magically stop eating and feel full when you are done. The best part is that fullness continues all the way through to lunch (or whatever your next meal is). No more eating your lunch at 10am after that bowl of oatmeal or breakfast yogurt leaves you hungry for more about half an hour later. Granted, there may be some high fat, high protein foods somewhere out there that may cause you to overeat, but I guarantee higher carbohydrate binge foods outnumber those by a long shot. Limit the latter to signal to your body that you are eating for nutrients and that it is full and you'll soon see improvements in regulating hunger, impulsive overeating and lack of self-control.

Yes, we all "cheat" sometimes when it comes to food. We all may also act like an impulsive third grader at times (myself included). The best strategy is to be controlled about it for the best end result. Choose foods that will reward you while satiating you: choose dark chocolate with a higher percent of fat and fiber versus milk chocolate with more sugar and less fat. High quality aged cheese will fill you up a lot faster than a plate of cookies. (As a side note, for the chocolate make sure the first ingredient is cacao beans or else you are likely eating chocolate liquor and not real chocolate. Also, check lists online or scour other available resources to ensure it is low in cadmium or lead, as some brands—including brands found at Whole Foods and other expensive health markets—can be high in both.)

Lastly, sometimes we just want to feel full from our cheat. Once again, choose "anti-binge" sessions with foods that don't make you want to eat more. This will allow you to defeat compulsive eating, setting yourself up for the win. If you cannot put a certain food down or crave more after consuming it, DO NOT have it in your house. Even something as "all-natural and healthy" as salted almonds can derail some people—be honest with yourself about the foods that make you lose control. Admit defeat, and rid your kitchen shelves, snack pantries and office desk drawers of them—out of sight, out of mind.

3

EATING ENOUGH: SATIATE DON'T RUMINATE

I hate counting calories, and I have ALWAYS hated counting calories. It is a Sisyphean task that oftentimes adds extreme difficulty and ambiguity to an area that is already challenging enough for many people. Secondly, not all calories are the same, especially when we consider body composition and the fact that weight on the scale tells us nothing about fat mass or muscle mass, i.e. the key indices for body composition. Strangely enough, to the die-hard calorie counters a bowl of ice cream is the same as a spinach and egg omelet, as long as they have the same calories. Weight Watchers even used points to replace calories, further illustrating their agnostic approach to assessing the quality of what we consume. Calorie counters oftentimes ignore the appetite-stimulating effects of certain foods and the blood sugar rollercoaster that follows. In my hometown, there was a

Rita's Italian Ice right next to the local Weight Watchers center, which was probably an astute business maneuver as they know their customers—just a little won't hurt! Even better, Rita's may be pure sugar water, but it is likely lower in calories than ice cream!

To further illustrate these underlying issues, let's do a calorie counting example using yours truly as the subject. I weigh about 190 lbs. and my resting metabolic rate is roughly 2,400 calories/day. I got the latter from the indirect calorimetry device at our Exercise Oncology Lab, though I am not sure how useful a number it is. Resting metabolic rate tells you how many calories we burn simply by being alive—i.e. how much gas your car burns just sitting there and idling, not by going for a ride or speeding down the highway. (As a side note, I am happy with my weight but am always trying to put on more muscle, as I am approaching that age where I will lose it if I do not fight hard to keep it on. Thus, I try to keep my body weight up as opposed to wanting to reduce it.)

For this example, let's say a week goes by and I can't find the time to exercise, but I still eat three meals a day. Based on my resting metabolic rate above; to simply remain the same weight (again, ignoring activity) I need to eat three meals of 800 calories a day. If we add in my exercise routine and the several miles per day that I walk, as well as the calf raises I do all day while dictating at my desk, I need significantly more food simply to fuel my basic cellular needs and the various muscle contractions throughout the day. But for the sake of a simplified example, let's ignore all that.

If I eat equal meals throughout the day, that would again leave me with 800 calories for breakfast. Some would argue breakfast is the lightest meal, while others favor the "Eat like a king for breakfast, a prince for lunch, and a pauper for dinner" approach. A common breakfast for many individuals who are just beginning at our sessions is a bowl of oatmeal and some fruit, one of the favorite and unchanging recommendations of nutritionists and dietitians over the past 50 years. Those who really "eat healthy" often consume fat-free yogurt with fruit for breakfast. The latter is a fan favorite for many as it requires zero preparation and simply popping a lid off of a plastic carton, but we will talk more about that in Chapter 8. If I was an oatmeal eater with some fruit and ate a massive amount of 2 servings (i.e. 2 cups), that would give me about 280 calories. Throw an easily accessed banana on top for another 120 calories and I will be hitting 400 calories for breakfast, along with about 90 g of carbohydrates, 10 grams of protein, and very little fat. We'll dig deeper into the implications of eating nearly 100g of carbohydrates first thing in the morning with little protein a little later, but for the sake of this exercise consider that this leaves us with a necessary 2100 calories between my next two meals to hit even for the day.

If I make it to lunch without eating again, a difficult task after a breakfast consisting of nearly 100g of carbs with little fat or protein, I might next decide to follow common dietitian advice by going with a grilled chicken breast salad. Assuming this is a big portion size with some olive oil on top, I will be consuming another modest 400-500 calories.

As I come down the homestretch, I will need to consume a 1,500-calorie dinner to simply break even for the day, and this again is not considering any activity. Also, keep in mind that our bodies have no choice but to abide by the law of homeostasis—they like to stay in the same metabolic state and will alter our cellular processes, our hunger, and even our mental and emotional states to keep it that way. If we under-eat, our metabolism will slow down. Try to throw in some exercise, and it will get worse. Adding further insult to injury, our body will likely throw hunger at us in an attempt to get our daily calories where they need to be. For some of us, this hunger can be ravenous and difficult to rein in.

Steve Phinney, a noted physician and metabolism researcher, took 12 overweight inpatients and cut their calories down to 720 per day; he observed their average metabolism rates drop by 10%. When he then added in a calorie-restricted exercise group to observe in parallel, he noted that their resting oxygen consumption dropped an additional whopping 17%. Interestingly, the groups lost a similar amount of weight due to the metabolic compensation for the cut calories and exercise.[2]

Long story short, with a paltry first two meals you are likely not going to hit your calories for the day, and your body is going to punish you for it. In the evening while you watch your nightly Golden Girls episodes, all of a sudden the hunger will start to hit, beckoning like a devil in your ear. Even worse, you will be dealt the challenge of satisfying this hunger by either consuming real food or simply grabbing readily available comfort food at arm's length. You've had a long day and the effort it takes to prepare a real food dish is beyond your comprehension at this stage. Worse yet, our body and our metabolism often challenge us as we are winding down after a long and stressful day of physical or mental activity. Fighting this hunger is a Sisyphean task for most of us, especially if we are struggling with stress at work, anxiety over all the possibilities to make us anxious throughout the day, and of course, those of us going through treatment for cancer have plenty to be anxious about. The next thing you know, you are eating a couple cookies here, a couple there, a small piece of chocolate, and a handful of potato chips every time Blanche and Rose trigger the sitcom laugh track. Before the episode credits roll, you've ended up getting those 2400 calories down, satisfying our body's push for homeostasis. Tucking yourself into bed, you realize your efforts to eat "healthy" backfired, as you ended up under-consuming protein for the day while carb-loading a gut-busting 300 grams. And here's the cherry on top of the carb-loaded sundae: the body is generally less able to efficiently process carbohydrates at night due to decreased insulin sensitivity, adding further fuel to the fire.[3]

And who are we kidding? You likely did not even make it through the day without snacking. Few of us can make it to those nightly hunger pangs, and instead we end up eating our lunch at 10am once our blood sugar from breakfast starts to drop (a frequent episode I encountered during medical school when I was eating a more "heart healthy" breakfast, or so they told me). Or, we simply pick all day at the plethora of junk food that our coworkers put on the break room table. In the very common example above, starting the day off by calorie counting and the reductionist approach of eating to minimize, as opposed to eating for nutrition (i.e. to maximize), may very well lead to far too many calories, far too little nutrition, and far too much hunger, all ending in disaster.

We need to set ourselves up to succeed. Countering the example above, let's suppose I wake up and eat 6 eggs for breakfast, thoroughly frightening every dietitian from sea to shining sea. Let's also suppose I throw in some onions, spinach and raw cheddar cheese made from the milk of grass-fed cows, and then cook it all up in some butter also from grass-fed cows. A dash of salt and pepper and if I'm feeling extra adventurous some Calabrian chilies will be sprinkled on top. Already I am hitting around the 700-800 calorie mark with this meal, along with around 40 or more grams of protein, 35 grams of fat, 8 grams of fiber, a handful of polyphenols and plant chemicals, anti-inflammatory conjugated linoleic acid, and an array of fat-soluble vitamins and minerals including calcium and vitamin K2. While this meal will provide ample fullness all the way through to lunch, there will be no blood sugar rollercoaster as nearly all the carbohydrates are fiber, as opposed to the prior breakfast which was around 10% fiber with the remaining carbohydrates digested as sugar. This meal also helps me hit my daily goal of protein to help maintain or increase muscle mass (the number to reach this goal is controversial and will be discussed shortly, but is generally around 0.6-0.8g per pound of ideal body-weight, or about 75% of your weight in grams of protein. The range should be generally on the higher end as we age, if we are attempting to lose weight, or are at risk for muscle loss due to a medical condition.

Returning to the above example, now add in a similarly nutrient-composed lunch made up of a bed of greens, some colorful vegetables, a protein/fat source, some olive oil, and perhaps even some blackberries. Voila—you have a similar high-calorie meal that is incredibly nutrient-dense and leaves you full until you get around to making a similar dinner. No snacking is necessary, and you eat dinner and then go to bed several hours later feeling full. In fact, if I find myself hungry at night, it tells me that I likely did not eat enough during the day, and I take note of that and adjust for tomorrow. Snacking during the day generally signals that meals are too small—fixing the meal size issue often fixes the snacking.

Ironically, a reductionist eating approach more often will leave me eating more for the day, as my body pushes to get adequate nutrition with mixed hunger signals. Taking the opposite approach and eating with the primary goal of obtaining adequate nutrition leaves me in a successful position as I navigate the day, particularly with the stresses of my work. Additionally, these meals are rich in polyphenols and other chemicals that stimulate my immune system to overcome the potential detrimental effects of stress.

In other words, a reductionist approach with respect to calories often plagues those individuals trying to keep the excess dietary fat and calories down as they end up not eating enough, particularly at breakfast. Having too much adipose tissue is most often the result of eating too much quantity and too little quality. To correct the issue, we need to focus on both sides of the coin, not merely the quantity side. Additionally, focusing on quality is required if we are eating for our health, which requires adequate nutrients, minerals and vitamins, along with well-sourced protein to build and repair from our cells to our organs.

One more friendly reminder that all of the above is assuming I am doing nothing but idling all day. In reality, I walk several miles per day, labor in the yard for several hours a week, chase my children around, and cycle between strength, conditioning and hypertrophy training regimens in the gym for 4-5 days per week. If I ate what we described above—an eating pattern that most dietitians promote—I would be ravenously hungry most of the day and even more so at night. I would "fail" their recommendations and habitually feel quite bad about myself. I would be unable to work out effectively and would have even more trouble maintaining muscle mass—forget about gaining any muscle—and recovering from those intense workouts. If you have tried the above exercise repeatedly and failed, you are not alone: the vast majority of us are destined to fail with that approach. If you instead turn toward eating for nutrition and quality, as opposed to reducing calories and fat, you may find in your new approach a path with less friction and a higher chance of success—one that leaves you with more energy and muscle mass and less anxiety and fat mass.

4

IGNORING THE AMBIGUITY: WORDS VERSUS REALITY

Whether you asked for it or not, somebody has very likely, and probably very recently, informed you of the merits of eating a plant-based or Mediterranean diet. They may not be able to clearly define what either of those terms mean—the Mediterranean covers a vast geographic area from Spain to Italy to Egypt—or even tell you what their diet exactly is, but they are more than happy to strongly advise that you follow them. I am often asked by my clients the question "Have you watched the Blue Zones documentary?" It highlights five areas throughout the world where the locals experience incredible longevity, including Okinawa, Japan, Sardinia, Italy, Nicoya, Costa Rica, Ikaria, Greece, and Loma Linda, California. This question is often followed by a vague discussion of a plant-based diet. I love to ask what the Greeks did with all those lambs and goats running around during the show. They must have had a lot of pets! Calorie counting—that impossible task—is another ambiguous favorite of the dietitians, along with the "exercise more and eat less" advice. The trapdoor to this "advice" is that it is almost always vague, undefinable, and thus impossible to follow. And that is the rub: when you, dear well-meaning dieter, end up gaining weight, the blame will be squarely on you as you didn't follow their "precise" directions! Nutritional advice has become incredibly adept at gas lighting those who seek it. Never mind that I, personally, may eat a plant-based diet and also a meat-based diet (or sometimes even a wine-based diet, depending how one defines it). The first thing I consume in the morning is coffee, so perhaps I follow a coffee-based diet? If you do not know what the heck your diet even means, you will likely fail at your goals. And when you fail, you will shoulder the blame.

With respect to the fad diet list above, the best strategy is to cast aside the vagueness and hone in on precision and simplicity. We eat for nutrition, not to prune plants or to follow in the footsteps of Italians, Greeks, Northern Africans, or any of our other societal brethren scattered about the Mediterranean Sea, particularly when those peoples, wise as they are, cannot and could not even accurately define what they put into their bodies. Those of us with actual families that come from the Mediterranean scoff at these online descriptions, particularly my boisterous grandmother who helped run her Italian grocery, made dozens of pounds of soppressata and sausage, cooked with lard and held regular "head cheese parties" (look it up) for her neighbors. For some strange reason dietitians have thoroughly embraced providing vague advice that is difficult to decipher, from counting those amorphous calories (impossible) to eating a plant-based diet (vague and confusing). The same dietitians will tell you that you need more protein but in the same breath say that you should only be eating plants, which are one of nature's least protein-infused food resources. To obtain adequate daily protein from plants alone, one would have to eat a nearly impossible amount of roots, leaves and stalks, directly violating their dietitian's advice to eat less. For instance, if I aimed to achieve an adequate amount of daily protein from "high protein" green beans, I would have to eat at least 11 pounds per day, and some would argue this should be closer to 18 pounds (see Chapter 5). And thus begins your circular jog on the hamster wheel, with no incremental results and no end in sight.

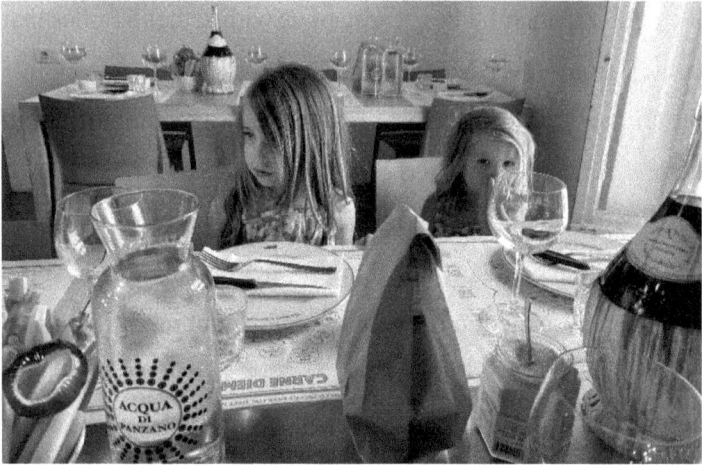

My daughters Aurelia and Chiara await their 7-course meat lunch at Dario Cecchini's in Panzano in Chianti. It includes all you can eat vegetables as well (and wine for the adults). Is this plant-based?

Some of my colleagues believe this to be some sort of sinister move, but I am not convinced of the malicious intent. Rather, I think it is both mental laziness and frustration with having to follow utterly incorrect (and borderline insane) guidelines that remain heavily influenced by the antiquated "Food Pyramid" and perpetuated by special interest groups. This house of cards was built in the 70s, and although modern nutrition science has killed it time and again, its mummy corpse continues to sleepwalk through our hallowed institutions, poisoning our views on health half a century later.

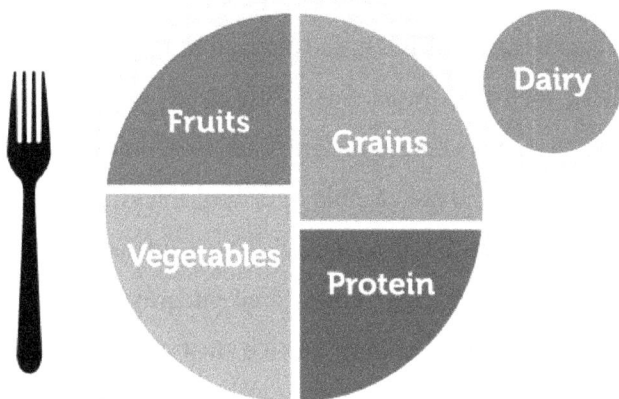

The "Food Pyramid" is heavily plant-based, with 10-12 servings of grains recommended per day—the same amount you would give to a cow to make it nice and fat before sending it to the slaughterhouse. In subsequent years this triangular terror has been replaced with several geometry-inspired derivations, and most recently Michelle Obama's pie chart food plate. As you look at it, pay no attention to The Who song "Won't Get Fooled Again" playing in the background:

Meet the new boss. Same as the old boss.

Unfortunately, we the public have been fooled again, and again and again. And a quarter of the way into the 21st century, the foolhardiness has shown no signs of stopping.

Dietitians and nutritionists are in a tight spot: they are still being taught this foolishness and directed by the powers above to advise such half-truths and full fallacies to patients, yet many have come to realize the grave issues in doing so. Those in the industry who are capable of critical thinking no longer want to participate in setting their clients up for disaster. Many have gotten sick of their professional integrity being called into question by providing advice that rarely produces successful results. Still others are in a more precarious position, where offering advice outside of the status quo may earn them a verbal reprimand or worse yet may cost them their job. "Stay in your lane!" the nutrition overlords say, one that avoids critical thinking and doesn't foster any societal improvement. Go on with the status quo even though it's failing; don't rock the boat. The latter attitude is what I feel is largely responsible for the prevailing advice. The ambiguity allows them to toe the line and avoid making those exact recommendations they are fully aware will lead to disaster, yet also not make ones that will get them into trouble with their bosses. As a result, clients in pursuit of healthy eating advice are often given conflicting information, such as to follow a plant-based diet while simultaneously consuming lots of protein.

The prevailing motivation for perpetuating this state of ambiguity that accompanies the Mediterranean Diet, the plant-based diet, etc., is that it places the onus on us, the dieters, when we fail. It's not the vehicles themselves that are ineffective, it's the drivers who are failing. They used to push impossibly low-calorie diets along with low-fat diets (a tough combination to follow); this has gradually segued to diets where it is not even clear what the diet actually is. "Plant-based" is generally a code word for "vegetarian" or even "vegan", yet many of us eat plenty of animal-based foods and perhaps even more plants. Is that "plant-based"? Then, why not just state "vegetarian" plainly and clearly? Well, because then the chance of failure becomes clearer, as everyone is aware of the difficulty of being a vegetarian.

Focusing upon the ambiguity exposes the main issue: we generally need animal-based foods to adequately nourish our bodies, stay healthy and achieve (and then maintain) our ideal weight. There are people who can accomplish these physiological objectives without consuming animals, but they constitute a very small minority of the general population, and even then only a subset of that minority can manage this difficult task with a reasonable amount of controlled precision. Furthermore, some believe that if we also avoid dairy, obtaining adequate nutrition becomes impossible. On the contrary, we can rely on foods like whole fat dairy to provide the necessary fat-soluble vitamins A, D, E, and K, along with conjugated linoleic acid. When this is fermented as cheese, we get some extra vitamin K2 to help pull calcium into our bones alongside vitamin D3. Arguably the consideration of greatest importance, especially in a cancer patient who has just finished a course of chemotherapy or anyone approaching middle age or later, is the importance of eating to avoid low muscle mass.

Humans need muscle mass to function physically, metabolically and cellularly. This is why women with more muscle mass have a greater chance of curing their breast cancer.[4] This is why pancreatic cancer patients with lower muscle mass have much lower odds of beating cancer back into remission.[5] Yet, if you listen to widespread nutrition advice for individuals during cancer treatment, or go to the American Institute for Cancer Research (AICR) website, it is all about plants—eat plenty of fruits, grains, and vegetables. Where does one get their protein? There isn't enough stomach space for the amount of beans needed to get in the required protein (let alone a GI tract strong enough to tolerate them.). Yet, the AICR recommendation on protein amount is silent. For instance, it tells us:

"In your blueprint to beat cancer, it helps to think of animal proteins like fish, poultry, and lean red meat as a complement to your mostly plant-based meals. Load your plate with greens and grains, and let meat be a secondary focus of your meal...

Don't feel like every meal you make has to include meat. Have fun exploring plant-based recipes, and enjoy some lunches and dinners that are entirely plant-based."

Besides the reductionist approach for protein above and the question mark as to whether one is able to get enough protein with this approach, notice how these recommendations trace back to the food pyramid. Also, notice the recommendation to avoid high protein foods, but instead "load your plate" with grains. Does this advice sound familiar—should we load it with perhaps 10-12 servings a day? Not to pick on the AICR, but they perfectly illustrate the confusion imparted on us by well-meaning nutrition and dietary recommendations, even from legitimate sources. Further down in their recommendation they show pictures of meal ideas, and one is a mix of tomatoes, onions, corn, zucchini and peppers in a serving size that resembles about 3 grams of fat, 3 grams of protein and 200 calories. How is one to nourish themselves and also provide adequate protein and calories through meals like this?

Words versus reality...

It is nearly impossible for any average-sized adult to subsist on such nutrient-sparse meals, let alone generate the energy to do anything worthwhile throughout the day. Are we simply setting up people for failure, anxiety and defeat by recommending meals that may lead to muscle loss and hunger? Do the creators of these meal plans actually follow them? Are they able to survive on a measly amount of protein, fat and calories?

I am dismayed by the infrequency with which today's nutritionists, dietitians and other health-promoting sources recommend animal-based foods, especially since these same authority figures mention with relative frequency why it is important to get adequate nutrients and protein. Meats and eggs are some of the most protein- and nutrient-dense foods, yet they seem afraid to recommend them—even to a cancer patient who is malnourished, protein-deprived and at massive risk of muscle loss, if not already cachectic. Instead, they will recommend ill-defined patterns like Mediterranean and plant-based diets, or contradictory approaches like getting adequate protein while loading your plate with grains.

There is certainly not one perfect eating pattern for everyone. However, individuals will often turn recommendations to ephemeral ambiguous dust. While these may be harder to argue with, there have to be some boundaries as to what is likely the best eating pattern for the majority of people. This is especially true considering what those of us in the medical field see in practice.

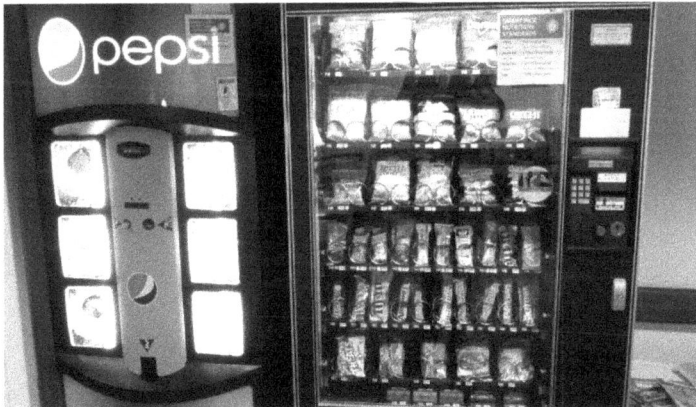

The above was taken from the waiting room of a cancer center, where we apparently go to receive healthcare.

This repeated violation of common sense is observed *ad nauseum* in the world of oncology, where patients undergoing various forms of cancer treatment are told the above but then in the very next breath offered donuts, cakes, cookies, pretzels and other grain and sugar-based sweets while undergoing chemotherapy (and are on high doses of steroids, which already raise blood sugar and reduce insulin sensitivity). Be that as it may, I will refrain from passing harsh judgment on those of my colleagues who harbor a soft spot for such sympathy treats... for now. And when we get to Chapter 7, we'll dig a bit deeper to see if these "grain good guys" and "sugar saviors" are as sinister as I've made them out to be.

5

Protein, Carbs, and Over and Under Eating

Generally speaking, at our Nutrition Sessions we encounter two main groups of individuals struggling with food intake: 1) those with excess adipose tissue, and 2) those who are extremely lean but possess too little muscle mass. Not everyone struggling with nutrition fits into these two categories, but the overwhelming majority do have one of these two aspects as their primary issue, and the attendance profile at our sessions corroborates this data. The second case type is less common, while the first case type is dominant and continues to increase in prevalence. Below are the rates of obesity in the US from 1999 to 2018, per the National Health and Nutrition Examination Survey conducted by the National Center for Health Statistics:

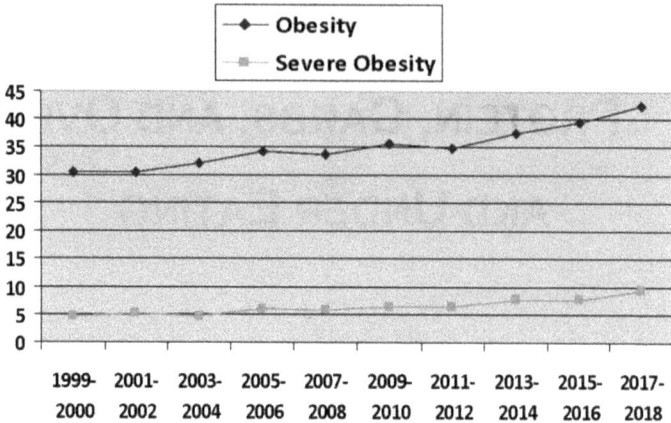

Obesity rates continue to climb in the wrong direction, with severe obesity creeping up as well over the past decade. The majority of individuals with too much adipose tissue generally consume too many carbohydrates—specifically sweets, processed carbs, bread, pasta and rice. While the calorie counters reading this may take issue with that comment, I am not stating that this group does not eat too many calories, as the two frequently go hand-in-hand. For instance, in the EXERT-BCN study I conducted in 2023-2024, we avoided any calorie counting and instead targeted reduction of carbohydrate-rich foods, focusing on eating high-quality nutrients, keeping carb levels under 100 grams per day, and optimizing protein intake at 0.6-0.8 grams per pound of ideal body weight. We met at regular intervals with the study participants to review their food choices, dissuading them from adding and subtracting meal quantities and portion sizes and encouraging them to focus on what foods comprised their meals, ensuring they were high quality and followed the above rules. Subjects ate a protein/fat with colorful and green leafy veggies at each meal, cut out grains, and went up or down on fruit based on their fat loss goals, in other words, what we always recommend for nutrition. The women that reduced their consumption of carbohydrates saw the greatest fat loss; several of these cases exceeded expectations to the point of straining credulity. One subject lost an incredible 27 pounds of fat in 3 months; the majority also lost some measurable amount of fat while gaining muscle, a product of our intense resistance training regimen for study subjects utilizing heavy weights and compound movements.

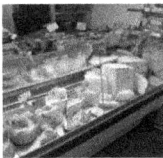

01
No calorie counting, eat nutrient-dense foods

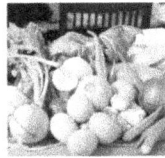

02
Limit processed foods, sugar, bread, pasta

03
Cook, eat with family, no snacking

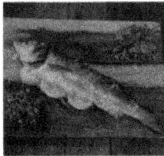

04
Quality>quantity : whole foods, grass-fed meat

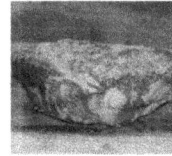

The above picture shows the 4 tenets of the EXERT-BCN study, promoting high quality foods.

Recalling our discussion in Chapter 2, high carbohydrate foods are drug-like in nature in that individuals have trouble controlling when to stop, leading to binge-like eating. These carb binges paradoxically leave their bingers feeling physiologically hungrier and emotionally in a state of self-loathing, particularly when occurring in isolation. This explains why endless bread baskets at "Italian" restaurants like Bravo and Olive Garden often leave diners feeling bad about themselves afterwards, and then hungry 30 minutes later when their blood sugar is on the downward drop of a roller coaster ride. For anyone who has proven they have struggled with overeating carbs and sugars in the past, keeping them as low on your personal "Rules of Eating" list and out of sight, out of mind is a prudent starting strategy. However, bear in mind that many individuals (including me) struggle with eating even the smallest amounts of these foods and thus avoiding them completely is the best strategy.

And what of the second face of our two-sided coin, those who are lean but with lower amounts of muscle mass? They often struggle with protein consumption, and for many this is the missing link in their diet. They have no issue overeating and frequently function like metabolic furnaces, burning through everything they eat. Interestingly, recent data suggest that only 40% of women eat the recommended daily amount (RDA) of protein.[6] The Dietary Reference Intake (DRI) recommends 0.8g per kg of body weight per day, or 0.36 g per pound ideal body weight. For a 150-pound lean individual, this would come to 54.5 grams per day. This recommendation constitutes the absolute bare minimum, yet top researchers and experts consider this number exceedingly low for anyone who wishes to preserve or build muscle mass. Furthermore, for those of us at risk of muscle loss (or sarcopenia)—which is basically every person past middle age, the point when we become generally less effective at turning dietary protein into muscle mass—we actually need to increase our protein consumption. Individuals losing weight for whatever reason also require more protein to avoid losing muscle mass. Lastly, we must once more ask ourselves, as we did in Chapter 3, what are we supposed to eat the rest of the day if the amount of protein equates to 218 calories?

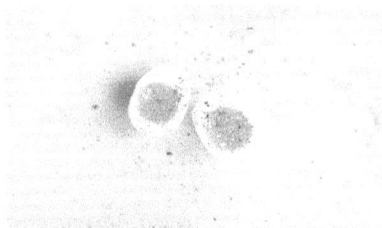

Increase
Protein:
0.6-0.8g/lb
per day

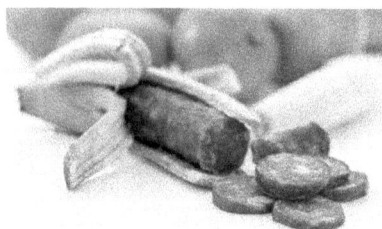

Keep
Carbs
under 100
g/day

In EXERT-BCN, we had individuals keep their carbs below 100 g/day to lose fat. The above protein amount was a goal as well (to achieve without counting), and with high-quality food choices, this was generally easy to meet.

Strangely, the DRI proposes that "No more than 25 percent of energy should be consumed as added sugars." They also recommend consuming it as 10-35% of our energy consumption. Here we should pause and ask ourselves: "Are they really recommending that we eat more sugar per day than protein?" I doubt that anyone on their committee would agree with that statement, but when you do the math, their own document can lead to that conclusion. Again and again, we see this gap in the recommendations—if we are told the erroneous advice of limiting fat and eating small amounts of protein, carbohydrates will logically fill the gap. Worse yet, added sugar will be part of this equation, which is oddly permitted for up to a quarter of our diet by the DRI. Given this anomaly, perhaps the obesity graphs at the beginning of this chapter are not so surprising after all. Could you imagine eating 25% of your daily calories in sugar? It is unclear how anyone not training for the Olympics could maintain a normal body composition at that rate, yet this is what is recommended in the official dietary guidelines. At the EOC, we recommend under 100 grams of carbohydrates per day for anyone trying to lose adipose tissue and individuals will go up or down in this number (mostly by eating fruit) based on their goals.

Bottom line: we need more protein than the DRI currently says that we do, especially because we should all be lifting weights with the goal of increasing or preserving our lean muscle mass. Additionally, stressing and damaging our muscles during workouts with heavy weights and adequate repetitions requires increased dietary protein, along with amino acids to repair the muscle fibers and preserve their integrity. Studies across the past several decades emphatically reinforce that weight training makes us more efficient at utilizing protein, and data from more recent studies reveal that our muscles utilize an extremely high amount of protein specifically after workouts, opening the door for those of us who struggle throughout the day to get enough protein.[7]

Putting an end to the willpower-testing habit of endless bread baskets at Italian restaurants is a wise health strategy applicable to all. In parallel, keeping high-protein foods high on your "Rules of Eating" list is a complementary strategy for every healthy eater.

6

AVOIDING THE SLIPPERY SLOPE

The *Golden Girls* evening reruns blocks are scheduled on your satellite dish service's "Classic TV Shows" channel for the umpteenth time this week, and after putting the kids to bed you are jonesing for some instant nostalgia to help you doze off. You stay up to watch a few episodes and once again end up watching several hours' worth while scrolling on your second screen, then make it from the couch to your bed just in time to get 7 hours of sleep—that is, of course, because you sprint like your hair is on fire from the time you wake up until you clock in to start your work day. A stress-inducing drive with a few speed limits broken awaits you as well as you scramble to get to the steel mill factory just on time. You may have thought you won the first leg of your daily race, but unfortunately, you've already lost. You, my friend, are a loser by virtue of having tumbled down the slippery slope.

The good news is that you only lost for that day. (And, perhaps any day after the hilarious geriatric hijinks of the *Golden Girls* were simply too good to stoke swift somnolence.) Why? You did not have time to make an adequate breakfast, so you streamlined some premade disaster at work or succumbed to grab-and-go on the way. It tasted good, but you felt terrible afterwards when your body realized you fed it junk to start the day, and your brain was confused as to why you fed it nutrient-sparse Soylent Green, signaling to it that today it would be a loser. You were hungry all morning, then you dove into the junk food stash your coworkers pick at almost every day while shrugging their shoulders and telling you they just can't seem to lose weight. You then washed that down with some premade salad that was sitting in the refrigerator bin at the coffee shop for four days staring at passersby, with its dried out and leathery lettuce drenched in rancid soybean oil sludge masquerading as olive oil. To your surprise (but not mine), this culinary crap also left you hungry and snacking all afternoon. Never mind going to the gym, as you already pounded down a solid day's worth of garbage and feel like… well, garbage. Now, that late-night binge session of Golden Girls appears to be the "gift" that just keeps on giving.

The good news for you here is that you have lots of chances to win and lose. In fact, all day long we can set ourselves up to be either winners or losers. Over the course of one's life there are finite games—games of skill (e.g. sports) and games of chance (e.g. cards), short-term games that are generally worthless in the grand scheme of things and can lead to greed, envy and lots of wasted time. Then, there are infinite games—those games with no end but of vital big-picture importance, like learning, striving for optimal health, embracing discomfort, living an intentional lifestyle, being good to others when no one is watching, etc. When we live an examined life—a life where we contemplate our actions, see the result of our actions, and reasonably question what we are told by others, society, the media, and our political "leaders"—we realize that playing the infinite game is the key to a fulfilling and successful life, and generally ignoring the finite games helps in this more noble pursuit. Additionally, the more insightful and disciplined of us realize that the finite games often lead us to spend more money, so those same sources that incorrectly tell us how to live our lives will nearly always push the finite games to trap us in the consumption cycle. (FYI, I would highly recommend reading the short book *Finite and Infinite Games* by James Carse.)

In reality, our work schedules surrounded by a multitude of non-work distractions and responsibilities can make simple things difficult enough. Thus, if we are not setting ourselves up for success (or avoidance of the disasters) we are setting ourselves up for disaster. For instance, if your job requires you to be at a desk all day, answer emails, create PowerPoints about nothing, sit in meetings to discuss future meetings where people use words like "granular" and "circle back" and just generally work in a cage-like existence, much effort is needed from the start to rewire this setup to make your existence more human. You need a standing desk, possibly a blue light if you have no window, a kettlebell to get some swings in during the day, lacrosse balls to roll out your feet, and certainly a prepared and filling lunch in some non-plastic containers to avoid the mouse feed hanging around the office.

Each day is a de facto Pavlovian response, starting from the second you wake up. Setting yourself up to win the day with a real, nutrient-dense breakfast that you created yourself signals to your brain that it is time to get going, and today we are going for the win. Much like Michael Jordan (or for you younger readers, Lebron James) clapping and spreading his hands through the air with baby powder before each game, your brain receives the signal loud and clear—it is "Go!" time. An instant nutrient-sparse Soylent Green breakfast does the exact opposite, signaling instantly available food, ultimate convenience, and oh don't you worry because minimal nutrients are needed to sit around all day and run on a half tank.

In other words, you lost right out of the gates. And you lost because you set yourself up for defeat. You told your body to lose, and it followed your directions. For instance, are you someone that binges each holiday and gains weight? Many Americans gain around a pound each holiday season going into the New Year and don't lose it afterwards. This is one of the strongest ways to set ourselves up for disaster to start the year. Some, if not all, of this weight accumulates throughout life, leading to substantial weight gain.[8] Such actions turn a time of celebration and being with family into self-sabotage.

Life is a series of wins and losses, of finite and infinite games. Are you setting yourself up for victory in the latter infinite game, or letting the former derail you? The good news is that you decide the games you play, and better yet, you are in control of the outcomes. You can set yourself up to be a winner.

Cultural and Traditional Safety Nets

Many cultural forces used to throw us a safety net, or better yet a rope to help us pull ourselves up from going over the slippery slope. The Golden Rules of religion, societal norms, cultural adages like i*kigai* in Japan, *arete* in Greece, and *fare bella figura* in Italy all tell us to take care of ourselves and be good people, *particularly* when nobody is watching. These age-old terms instruct us to be our best, work hard, be kind to others, and keep a fit figure. The latter obviously has deeper meaning than to look and dress nicely, but anyone who has been to Italy or grew up in the States near a traditional Italian community understands the deeper meaning. It is similar to why my grandmother's father would tell her, "We may be poor, but outside of the home we should be generous to others as if we are rich." Taking care of yourself meant you were part of the community.

How we act counts. Traditional societies and religions tell us we should care for ourselves and others, be ethical and moral when nobody is looking (*arete)*, and always give our best at life (*ikigai*). When consumerism spread around the US at lightning-speed, things seemed to change. This highly infectious virus told us to throw these old-fashioned sayings to the side, as anything modern was hip and anything old was passe. You can purchase whatever you need, and the more you purchase the better. And when all those bills from over-consumption add up and cause anxiety or even depression, just consume some extra healthcare and ask for some pills or potions from your doctor to fix that too. The only way out is by consuming more. Tomorrow can fix the ailments we caused today, especially with a little help from technology. While the progressive technocrats will cry out this mantra to most modern self-imposed issues, rarely does this strategy actually work.

This strategy is of course a recipe for disaster, a disaster that has been quite visible all around us as rates of obesity, diabetes, anxiety and depression—all byproducts of over-consumption—continue to rise even though supposedly our quality of life is going up. This is the slippery slope, and it is a tough one to traverse once you find yourself teetering on the edge. Worse off, in our present society you are guaranteed to find yourself on the slippery slope, particularly since we are forced onto it at an early age. Don't believe me? Watch 15 minutes of children's programs on TV. The commercials ram consumerism down their throats: toys, candy, fruit snacks and junk food. It is one of the first things they see during arguably their most impressionable period of life. An African proverb tells us:

"Mix yourself with the grain and you will be eaten by the pigs."

While this specifically refers to the company we keep, our society instructs us to mix with the grains from day one, training us to plunge over the slippery slope. In fact, avoiding that slippery slope becomes an unavoidable challenge in life. A walk through the grocery store or a drive through a local strip mall reveals all we need to see—there is no principle of *bella figura* or *arete* pushing us to be better people. Instead, there are aisles upon aisles of processed junk options barely resembling food goading us into over-consuming. The utter lack of *ikigai* or being your best self is palpable. The resulting health issues are not medical problems "fixed" with medical consumption or the latest phone app, as they start well before a trip to the doctor and poke deeper at the core of our modern society. Falling over the slippery slope of consumerism and then consuming more medical care only worsens the problem as we again tell our brain that we can buy our way out of our issues. If we curtail our consumerism, limit excesses and take responsibility for our actions, we will reposition ourselves on a fast track to both mental and physical betterment.

Unfortunately, the slippery slope is all around us. Television and handheld devices often push us over the edge by keeping us up late at night, distracted and nonproductive in those parts of life that matter. Something as simple as eating premade meals in the morning or eating in our car pushes us over the edge as it tells our brain food is an instantly ready pleasure, a quickly consumable plastic container of dopamine, not an important source of nutrition that fuels our body and we must thus put in some effort to prepare properly. Packaged foods quickly leave us sliding down that slippery slope.

The slippery slope is a dangerous place requiring all of our intestinal fortitude to avoid sliding down and even more effort to get back onto solid footing. In our EXERT-BCN study, we mandated that all participants eat cooked meals with family and friends, never in the car or in front of the television. We also asked that participants avoid premade and packaged foods, curtail snacking, and push to eat real food. We recommended they eat about 70 grams of protein per 100 pounds of ideal body weight and limited their carbohydrates to under 100 grams. Interestingly, when you push towards real food and cooking, those changes in macronutrients are easy to achieve. We did not have participants calculate anything out, we just had them fill out food frequency questionnaires once a month and reviewed it with them. We also had our biweekly nutrition sit-downs.

In other words, we pushed *fare bella figura*, *ikigai*, and *arete*. We pushed for participants to return to viewing food as food. Additionally, we had everyone on study pull from the slippery slope together, like a herd migrating to better pastures. It is not surprising to learn that when individuals with cancer join an exercise program, the biggest factors that correlate with increased adherence and outcomes are: (1) doing it in person with others who hold you accountable and (2) training utilizing a prescription delivered by an expert.[9] Surrounding ourselves with motivated individuals has an immense effect on our effort in the gym, a point which has been underscored repeatedly when it comes to the cancer patient population.

In the famous words of Jim Rohn, "you are the average of the five people you spend the most time with." Rohn succinctly may have said what we all know deep down inside, but Miguel de Cervantes Saavedra beat him to the punch in the 1600s when he wrote in *Don Quixote*:

"Tell me your company, and I will tell you what you are."

In other words, it is not a newfound secret that if you are not surrounding yourself with positive, supportive nurturing friends who can help you grow and achieve the health you seek, it is time to find new friends or limit your interaction with the negative ones or bad influences. That is the unfortunate, but brutal, truth. However, you can't pick your work colleagues. So don't be surprised if you have those individuals at work that are always bringing in bagels, donuts and other nutrient-sparse addictive foods that make you feel terrible after, and do not be surprised if they try to force them on you. Also, do not be surprised if that is the same person always telling you they want to lose weight, but just can't get the pounds off. Unfortunately, many individuals would rather derail your health than use your positive changes to motivate themselves to improve. The latter takes effort and an admission that what one is currently doing may not be working. Additionally, many aspects of current society and the modern workplace promote envy instead of mimicking the masters in our lives—we can honor and try to imitate the brilliancy of Michelangelo, or we can try to tear down his masterpieces. Newsflash: we are all Michelangelos in one way or another, and good friends can promote our brilliant qualities, while bad friends can tear those same positive qualities down and build the negative ones up. It is up to you to surround yourself with a positive environment. This is a challenge for us all, but keep your eye on the prize and push ahead with your goals. Knowing that some individuals simply do not want the best for you and are trying to derail your efforts can be empowering as you push to overcome obstacles in life, even if those obstacles are a well-meaning neighbor consistently bringing pizza to your house and trying to talk you into eating it.

7

OATMEAL: THE WORST FOOD EVER (JOKING, KIND OF)

As we have discussed above, a majority of individuals in the United States struggle with poor body composition from having too much adipose tissue. Many of these individuals also complain about feeling hungry throughout the day, sometimes eating their lunch around 10am and often snacking at work in between breakfast and lunch and after lunch until the end of the day. As discussed in Chapter 3, many of these individuals "toe the line" at breakfast thinking they are going to cut calories to start the day, which hopefully will set them up to end the day with a net negative calorie count. While we have already discussed why this is very likely a failing strategy, examining more closely the foods that people often eat to start their day provides additional interesting insights.

Some people simply skip breakfast, and there is nothing wrong with that in general—though I would advise to avoid doing this too often, particularly if you are trying to maintain or gain muscle mass. Others use breakfast as a time to start the day by cutting calories, and still others use it to "carb load" with dessert-like meals (e.g. pastries, grains and donuts), derailing themselves before the day begins. When I ask my clients what they eat for breakfast, the most common responses are yogurt with fruit (nearly always the fat-free variety), a protein shake or protein-infused breakfast bar, or oatmeal with fruit. With the exception of some forms of oatmeal, I have noticed that these and most breakfast options are instantly made foods that require no planning or effort, which is an idea that has been foreign to the Homo sapiens species for about 99.9997% of our 300,000-year existence. We will come back to this later.

The oatmeal answer—not garnished with sugar, honey or other common taste-enhancing confections—nearly always comes from individuals that are earnestly attempting to be healthy, because it is a favorite recommendation by the medical establishment. When clients dig deeper and ask what makes oatmeal healthy, the follow-on response received is "fiber." OK, let's dig down one more layer. Our rational next questions are "How much daily fiber do we need?", and "Is oatmeal a good source of fiber?" In comes our old nemesis the DRI recommending 28 grams per day, if we're inclined to listen to it. So, does that make oatmeal a good source of fiber? We will answer that question in a moment, but the question we really are trying to answer for practical purposes is whether oatmeal is filling, particularly for those individuals having trouble getting all the way to lunch. The answer to the former question will explain the latter.

A single serving of oatmeal is a half-cup before adding water, and we can assume most people are eating a cup at breakfast. For plain oatmeal, this provides 5 grams of fat, 10 grams of protein, 56 grams of carbohydrates and 8 grams of fiber. Is almost 60 grams of carbohydrates a good cost to get 8 grams of fiber? Back in my on-the-go medical school days, 60 grams of carbs at breakfast via oatmeal was largely responsible for me consuming every lunch I packed for the long days by 10 am, including the protein or cottage cheese I would often add to the mix. The total carbohydrate count was so incredibly high that I would inevitably crash shortly after breakfast and need to consume something else to rescue me from the energy free-fall. This same experience is a common issue among the individuals in our Nutrition Sessions. Additionally, if you are attempting to ingest adequate protein, vitamins and minerals for the day, relying on those macronutrients will likely set most of us back, particularly for those of us sensitive to high carbohydrate diets. Almost certainly, 60 grams of carbs to start the day will have already tipped us over the tolerance scales, particularly if we are trying to lose weight.

The other more telling sign within the breakfast conversations is how many of the foods discussed can be heated up in a microwave or are readily available in a plastic container. Let's be honest: for many of us that is the real reason we eat yogurt, fruit, protein shakes/bars or oatmeal. The impetus has less to do with health and more to do with these foods being quick and easy, and if we are running late in the morning, they won't set us back from arriving at our jobs on time to settle into our cycle of sitting in endless meetings and "circling back" via emails. And this all points to a deeper issue regarding our relationship with food, one that signals that this relationship may not be in good form and thus requires retooling and/or rebooting. Likening this situation to a one-on-one romance or friendship, we might be "using" food as opposed to nurturing, deepening and expanding what we get out of it.

"But you just told me you are hungry all morning and can rarely get through to lunch." This is a comment you will hear me utter tirelessly in our Nutrition Sessions meetings. Almost without fail, the same individuals who overeat throughout the day due to their hunger lo and behold eat a nutrient-sparse breakfast with oatmeal as their typical breakfast. While oatmeal is frequently recommended as a good source of fiber, some sources even go as far as citing oatmeal as a good source of protein. Looking at the chart below, would you consider oatmeal to be a prudent decision, a good trade, when it comes to "the cost" of procuring those couple grams of protein? In fact, many foods touted as good sources of protein turn out to be less than optimal when we visualize the baggage that come with them when considering non-fiber carbohydrates:

Food	Total Carbohydrates (g)	Fiber (g)	Fiber:Carb Ratio
Long Grain Rice	45	0.6	0.01
White Bread	54	3	0.06
Millet	41	2.3	0.06
Quinoa	40	5.2	0.13
Whole Wheat Bread	42	5.7	0.14
Oatmeal	**56**	**8**	**0.14**
Sweet Potato	24	3.8	0.16
Bell Pepper	7.5	1.3	0.17
Beans	54	10	0.19
Rye Grains	128	26	0.20
Eggplant	49	14	0.29
Tomato	4.8	1.5	0.31
Kale	7.3	2.6	0.36
Carrot	11.4	4.2	0.37
Broccoli	3.6	1.7	0.47
Almonds	7	3.6	0.51
Okra	14.4	8	0.56

The above chart makes a clear case that not only is around 60 grams of carbs—and first thing in the morning!—a bad trade-off for 8 grams of fiber, but, as you will see below, it is an even worse trade-off for protein. We have great need for protein both when we are exercising and resistance training (which we all should be doing) and also as we age and thus are at risk of loss of muscle mass, reduced strength and range of motion, and even sarcopenia. Moreover, conducting similar analysis with respect to the nutritionist directive to consume oatmeal and other plant proteins once more reveals math that doesn't quite add up. This analysis is critical at present since we are being told left and right that we can get all our protein from plants or by following a plant-based diet (whatever this actually means—recall my rant in Chapter 4). Reviewing the protein amounts in the table below, would a plant-centric diet enable you to get enough daily protein to adequately support your body, cells, and muscle mass?

Food	Total Carbs (g)	Fiber (g)	Protein	Protein:Carb Ratio
White Bread	54	3	3.3	0.06
Carrot	11.4	4.2	1	0.09
Long Grain Rice	45	0.6	4.3	0.10
Sweet Potato	24	3.8	2.3	0.10
Eggplant	49	14	4.7	0.10
Quinoa	40	5.2	4.1	0.10
Okra	14.4	8	1.5	0.10
Rye Grains	128	26	17	0.13
Millet	41	2.3	6.1	0.15
Oatmeal	**56**	**8**	**10**	**0.18**
White Bread	54	10	12	0.22
Tomato	4.8	1.5	1.1	0.23
Whole Wheat	42	5.7	12	0.29

Bread				
Bell Pepper	7.5	1.3	2.2	0.29
Broccoli	3.6	1.7	1.2	0.33
Kale	7.3	2.6	2.5	0.34
Almonds	7	3.6	7	1.00

Additionally, would the cost be worth it? For instance, to obtain 15 grams of protein from black beans, you would need to consume 40.8 grams of carbohydrates. Attempting to utilize beans to achieve the adequate protein amount to support our muscles would require a massive dose along with a large amount of carbs. Setting aside the severe impact this would have on your gastrointestinal tract, is a reliance on beans even remotely feasible for adequate protein consumption for the majority of the population? Returning to oatmeal, one would have to consume over 110 grams of carbohydrates to obtain 20 grams of mediocre quality protein. Are the calorie counters obsessed with quantity comfortable with that trade-off? I know that I personally would balloon in weight by taking that approach, so I am certainly not comfortable providing this same recommendation to others, let alone those individuals trying to shed excess fat or attempting to maintain an optimal body composition.

Yes, I have singled out oatmeal as this chapter's villain and am picking on it to emphasize the issues above. However, if you are one of the rare individuals who finds ways to obtain adequate protein and nutrients and also consumes oatmeal without becoming ferociously hungry two hours later, then more power to you. (Still keep in mind that 60 grams of carbs in one little dish of oatmeal is quite high.) Yet for the rest of us—the overwhelming majority of society—this oft-cited breakfast choice perfectly illustrates the inherent issues with calorie counting, along with a misguided fear of fat and protein and the mental gymnastics people perform to convince themselves they can achieve adequate vitamins, minerals, nutrients and especially protein from plant-centric or other reductionist diets.

8

SABOTAGE!

PLEASURE FOODS OR PAIN FOODS?

During our nutrition discussions in "The Pit" I frequently hear about my clients' friends, family members, coworkers and even acquaintances or strangers consistently pulling them in the direction of eating foods that will derail their health efforts. In a strange and twisted way, a fair amount of people seem to take slightly perverse pleasure in watching other people engage in activities that are bad for their health. Perhaps it makes these individuals feel good about their poor choices, or at least less bad about them. Sounds twisted, huh? Unfortunately, it is rampant, particularly in medicine, and is probably a fundamental element of human nature. I hear about it all the time and watch it happen firsthand. And every time it does, I repeatedly hear as the soundtrack to these encounters the booming voice of the Beastie Boys screeching in the background:

"Listen all-a-y'all, it's a sabotage!"

The Grammy-winning American trio's 1994 rock-rap smash hit still resonates with the "Get Fit!" and "Pump You Up!" crowds around the world three decades later, and at the EOC you'll hear it several times a week during client workouts tied to their Nutrition Sessions. It's a surefire high-energy track that gets a good number of active participants (and staff!) going since the day we launched our facility. Not surprisingly to a geriatric millennial like yours truly, the Beastie Boys have a timeless gift for pumping everyone up from septuagenarian Baby Boomers to toddler Gen Alphas.

Music has a way of etching indelible memories onto one's mind, and I have my own fitness-related Beastie Boys story to share. Back at the turn of the century when I was an undergraduate student, I spent a decent amount of time at the university gym (no surprise) and "Sabotage" was a top tune on the "Workout Playlist" burned disc I toted around in my portable CD player. (Anyone born after 1999, feel free to Google "burned disc" and "CD player" please.). During my junior year, a younger member of my fraternity—let's call him Joe—approached me and asked if he could be my workout partner. Joe was a funny guy and we got along well, and his work ethic produced incredible gains. I was several years ahead of Joe in the weight room, but he progressed rapidly to close the gap and catch up to me—so much so that any time Dennis, our fraternity's resident chef, made one of his trademark desserts or stocked a new box of Chipwich ice cream cookie sandwiches (yes, these things exist and they are a full week's worth of anti-nutritional garbage packed into each serving), Joe would bring them to my room, dangle them in front of my face and goad me into trying to eat them. I would hear footsteps approaching, followed by Joe popping his head through my cracked door and teasing me in his cackling voice: "Coooooolin, don't you want one? They are delicious." Joe was committed to derailing my nutrition goals so that he could catch up with me.

While Joker Joe's jester antics were always lighthearted and good for laughs, this kind of diet and healthy lifestyle peer pressure does occur often in the real world. Instead of trying to build others up, we tear them down to match our internal hollowness. Instead of trying to mimic those masters in our lives, we would rather see if we can derail those around us to set them upon our lesser, slower-moving path. Sometimes the offers for desserts or junk food from others may come from a well-meaning place, but more often than naught we should stand our ground, taking our cue and inspiration from the Beastie Boys song lyrics:

"I can't stand it. I know you planned it!"

1. A patient receiving chemotherapy with high-dose steroids, artificially putting her blood sugar in a diabetic state was offered cupcakes and cookies by the infusion team... Sabotage!

2. Nutritionists telling overweight individuals to keep counting calories, cut fat and eat a bunch of foods that leave them hungry all day long... Sabotage!

3. People giving cookies, cakes and other sweets to individuals trying to lose weight... Sabotage!

4. Friends and family members telling you repeatedly, "Just this one time!" when you know it will absolutely not be just one time... Sabotage!

5. Academic exercise researchers and physical therapists telling you to resistance train at home using 2-pound weights, then writing dozens of negative papers describing the results... Sabotage!

6. Walking into a not-to-be-named local maternity hospital lobby and the first thing you see is a group of women at a table selling cookies and fudge of every flavor when everything a woman eats during pregnancy goes to the developing fetus... Sabotage!

7. Vending machines owned by Coke and Pepsi selling sugar water and candy at our government-run, taxpayer funded hospitals[9]... Sabotage!

"You'll shut me down with a push of your button

But, yo, I'm out, and I'm gone."

There is a litany of examples like the above illustrate why it is so vital to surround yourself with positive people that push you to be a better person (to yourself and to others) instead of continually coordinating efforts to derail and sabotage you. Keeping it together is hard enough when we have people supporting us, and nearly impossible when those around us engage in direct and indirect sabotage of our best-laid plans. While we strive to avoid the squirrels, ignore the naysayers, surround ourselves with beautiful people, places and things, and ignore the ugliness, still we often cannot avoid our family members and work colleagues. However, we can at least be honest with ourselves about the twisted efforts of those we see most frequently. While this all may sound cynical, we know it's true and very present in our lives, and as the saying goes: "The best offense is a good defense."

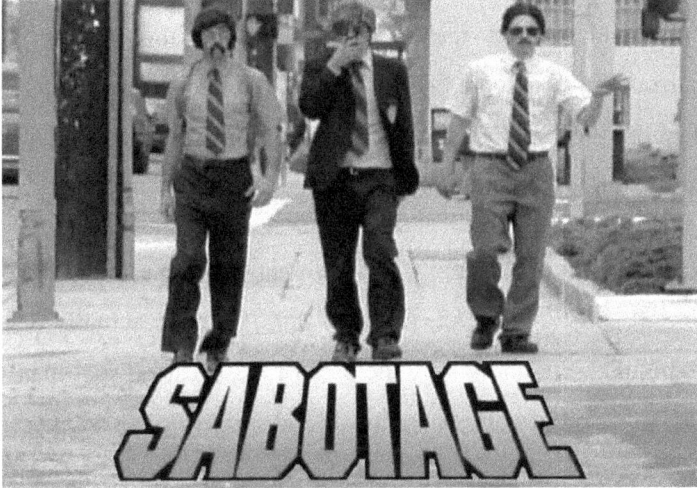

Sabotage remains a top 500 song of all time by *Rolling Stone* magazine. Little did the Beastie Boys know that their hit would predict a major future issue standing in the way of health.

Giorgio Vasari wrote books praising the masters of his time and Plutarch wrote about the character of the greats of antiquity. Nowadays, if you want quick notoriety, you put people down on social media. A famous popular example from my childhood was when professional figure skater Tanya Harding hired a hitman to take out the knee of her skating nemesis Nancy Kerrigan. If you can't beat them, then beat them down! Modern day gladiators are all around us, those who make their living beating others down. These modern-day gladiators focus more on the mental and emotional attacks these days. We have the choice of surrounding ourselves with saboteurs or positive promoters. Just don't expect hospitals or those giving you dietary advice to be full of the latter and free of the former.

While I am not necessarily saying these individuals are all sinister—in fact, you may think they are actually just being pleasant and taking the path of least resistance—many do have a bit of hollowness inside and simply do not want you to be "better" than them. This, of course, includes being more healthy and physically fit. The best thing we can do is to simply quit engaging in their bizarre competition, ignoring their finite game and instead focusing on playing the infinite games of life. Just as there will always be a devil on one shoulder, you will find an angel on the other: our sit-down sessions at the EOC are full of positive, nurturing individuals that strive to help those around them and motivate one another to stay on track. I am lucky enough to be an integral part of these sessions, and I routinely glean first-hand benefits from the infectious, positive nature of these individuals. The questions you must ask yourself are whether you are surrounding yourself with the same type of people, and whether their actions are trying to help you or sabotage you.

The next time you recognize someone trying the latter, I urge you to heed the advice of the Beastie Boys, play their unforgettable tune in your head and sing the words out loud if you must:

"What could it be, it's a mirage... You're scheming on a thing, that's SABOTAGE!!!!"

9

IT TAKES EFFORT

Everything worthwhile in life takes effort to achieve. Everything. And the good things often take even more effort. You may meet the perfect spouse—your soul mate sent down from our creator just for you, perfect in every way. Yet, a lifetime with this perfect person will still take plenty of effort. Staying healthy, sane, happy and fulfilled while minimizing stress, anxiety, depression and conflict takes unending effort. While this may seem Sisyphean at times, remember that this doomed mythological Greek's task of rolling his boulder back up the hill for eternity was both laborious and futile. The effort required to earn the best things in life may seem laborious at times, but it is not futile.

Getting enough sleep takes effort, and ideally you should be getting 8 hours a night (or maybe more in the winter). If not, ask yourself why. Walking, sleeping and breathing are required components of life. These background activities are non-negotiable. Stopping them leads to a quick or quicker death. Hunting and gathering real, nutritious food and then cooking it is a basic premise of life. It illustrates the importance of giving wholesome sustenance to our brain each and every time we engage in these activities. Prior to the mid-20th century, never in our history did we present ourselves with instant food premade for us with no effort. Never.

Giving our body a nutrient sparse (but low-calorie!) microwaved bowl of oatmeal in the morning is physically confusing for both our bodies and minds. A nutrient-dense meal that we produced through some effort tells our muscles and cells that it is "go time" and today is the real deal. It reiterates that food is so utterly vital, you planned ahead and went to bed at a reasonable time to wake up and prepare it. Staying up late from watching TV or playing on your device, thus forcing you to eat a premade breakfast while driving in your car, tells your brain the exact opposite. Even full-fat yogurt, which is a much better choice than that oatmeal, leaves us on our tippy-toes balancing on the precipice of a slippery slope. I have found that individuals who eat yogurt for breakfast are most of the time doing so out of convenience, out of not having their night before in their control such that they can wake up at the necessary time to start their day off correctly.

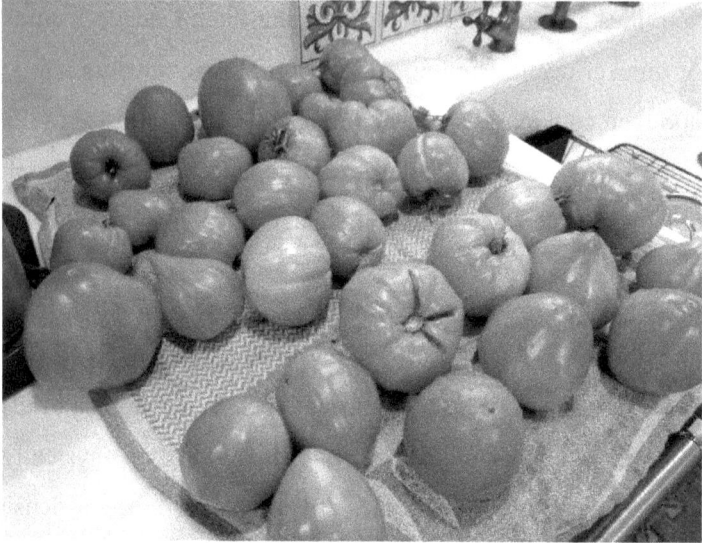

Yearlong planning and countless hours of effort and meditative gardening provide us with tomatoes and daily caprese salads every summer and fall.

More often than not, food choices mirror effort choices. If the effort is not there to start, forget about the food part of the equation because you have already failed. Every day is a competition—not just with your family members, friends and coworkers. Remember, every day is a competition with yourself. And if you are lacking the effort to compete, you start the day by losing. You have the choice to set yourself up for success each day. And you have the choice to remove those obstacles. You can turn off the WIFI or get rid of the devices that derail your efforts every day. You have the effort to empty your pantry and fill your fridge with real foods that need to be prepared. You have the determination to stop making excuses and stop blaming your situation on everyone and everything else.

But it takes effort. The good news is that effort is absolutely required in life, and with effort comes reward. Yes, remaining healthy in the 21st century is a Sisyphean task— the second we stop pushing that giant stone up the hill, it rolls right back down leaving us at square one. While remaining healthy is always a challenge, we live in a society controlled by large corporations and political groups that consistently pull the levers behind the curtain to inform us of our major issues (or even promote them…or even make up new ones altogether). Furthermore, these puppeteers dupe us into believing such issues can only be resolved by buying more of their products, supporting their groups, downloading the latest app, or following the latest "influencer" who coincidentally always seems to push some products or trendy diet. And worse yet, many societal and cultural stop gaps that historically kept us in check (e.g. religious-based temperance) have been called passe and removed.

Be that as it may, the results of this consumerism-driven society have repeatedly shown us that being healthy requires a lot more than following some vague or fashionable diet, and we just can't consume our way out of bad habits. Putting ourselves and our health first requires a lot more than putting on some trendy body shaping outfit or toting around a Lululemon bag and matching smoothie on the way to yoga class. Smoothies, superfoods, journaling and meditation apps won't do it either. These superficial attempts may be a product of the desire to be healthy, but we have to dig a lot deeper than surface image if we want to be successful. First and foremost, we must care.

And a realization of just how much we have to care to remain healthy sheds light on the humbling reality that all things in life that are meaningful and worthwhile are Sisyphean tasks. That's the rub, or exciting part depending on how you view it. We love our kids, but parenting them requires an immense amount of nonstop effort and a constant ride on an emotional roller coaster. We love our spouses, yet fostering a solid, dependable and even exciting relationship with them takes an incredible amount of unending work and compromise. We tend gardens of the figurative and literal varieties, which requires daily assessment, watering, pruning and weeding. The list goes on and on for those elements of life that make life worth living; they all require an immense amount of caring.

Our health is no different. In fact, our health may be most difficult because it requires caring while nobody is looking, little to no outside forces holding you accountable, and the constant bucking of the invisible hand of a consumerist society obsessed with politics and a raging, roaring "healthcare" machine. This society constantly pushes us to overdo it on the regular and then be "saved" by consuming its products, a major one being medicine in the form of pills, potions, and procedures.

When we boil it down to the basics, our health absolutely requires (in order):

1. Caring: Caring enough to want to maximize our health and be our best

2. Thinking: Critically thinking about ourselves, our actions, the environment around us, and how to grow

3. Action: Actually carrying out the necessary steps, without cutting corners

Without these three guiding principles, the finite games of back-and-forth, yoyo-ing diets, New Year's resolutions and other silly moonshots to achieve health result in a series of frustrating and unsuccessful superficial attempts. No overpriced pair of plastic stretch pants will overcome a lack of caring, critically assessing oneself, and taking action. In fact, more often than not, taking the route of over-consuming will only serve to fuel and worsen the underlying issues—issues that when properly addressed, alleviate the need for attempting to consume our unhealthy problems away.

As a side note, we often conflate motivation with caring—we can be motivated in many different ways. For example, we may be motivated to clean the yard, motivated to be good parents and motivated to get to the gym. But deep down inside, do we care? Motivation is kerosene that gets dumped on the fire of caring, but that initial flame must already be ignited. The former fuels all sources of the latter. When deep down inside we care, the actions and the lifestyle necessary to improve our health naturally precipitate: motivation to cook, eat well, remain active, lift heavy weights, ignore those around us that want to derail our health to feed their inner demons, get quality sleep, and put down our "digital cigarettes" (devices). These are no longer Sisyphean chores, but rather a normal and enriching part of our day. When we care, the questions change from "How do I get 8 hours of sleep a night?" to "Why wouldn't I get 8 hours of sleep a night?!?"

Things that were once excuses—but I have work, my kids get in the way, etc., etc.—only fuel us to push harder and be healthier. We'll work around our job schedule or take workday breaks to pursue healthy choices. Children will push us to be healthier so that we can be more active and more engaged parents. When stressed, we'll dig down deeper within ourselves to ensure we fuel our health. Unlocking these levels is when we have mastered the infinite game: a life of health and accomplishment, prior excuses now strengthening our conviction and further reiterating the importance of a healthy lifestyle that respects our body, soul, and mind. This is what caring fuels, and then it is manifested into reality by constant critical thinking and action.

"How can you pass on the cookies sitting on the table in the break room?" becomes "Why would I ever torture myself with those cookies or purposefully feed my body something that will make it look, feel, and function terribly?" The infinite game of caring trumps all the silly finite games that monopolize so much of our time. When we care and critically think, it becomes much easier to excuse ourselves from the silliness—our actions begin to reinforce to ourselves how much we care. We begin to enjoy pushing that boulder up the hill constantly—the Sisyphean task becomes the fulfilling task as it exercises our mind and body, sharpens our focus and purifies our purpose.

If we aim to be healthy and feel and function our best—and live a fulfilling life, I would argue—then caring, thinking and action are constantly required. Otherwise, individual health management turns into a precarious game with a slippery slope that we are likely to lose at despite our well-meaning efforts.

10

SUPPLEMENT ROUNDUP

When I published the first version of *Misguided Medicine* in 2014, I dedicated an entire chapter to the importance of avoiding supplements, and instead getting our vitamins, minerals and nutrients from actual food. I still stand by this overarching view, but I have also come to realize that this approach is not always possible in practice. For instance, what if our actual food simply did not contain the quantity or quality of nutrients it has in the past? Or, what if there was a disruption to our quality food supply chain? Unfortunately, this has proven to be the case with our modern food supply as of late. We constantly hear about how we are now living in the most technologically advanced society ever, yet we cannot even grow foods as nutritious as those that were grown during my grandfather's era.

For instance, a landmark study published in 2004 compared the nutritional content of 43 fruits and vegetables grown in 1999 versus 1950.[10] The results were not encouraging, as the researchers found significant declines in the content of protein, calcium, iron, phosphorus, riboflavin (vitamin B2) and ascorbic acid (vitamin C). When asked about their findings, the authors felt that the decline was due to agricultural practices that aim to increase crop size, yield percentage and resistance to pests and disease, as opposed to growing crops to increase nutrition. In other words, the plague of consumerism had found its way into our farms. The researchers also stated that "efforts to breed new varieties of crops that provide greater yield, pest resistance and climate adaptability have allowed crops to grow bigger and more rapidly, but their ability to manufacture or uptake nutrients has not kept pace with their rapid growth."

Donald Davis, the study's primary author, postulated that there were also likely decreases in magnesium, zinc, vitamins B-6 and vitamin E within produce from then to now. However, these latter nutrients were not studied in 1950, so he and his team were unable to compare them. Subsequent studies have reconfirmed the conclusions obtained by Davis and his food research teams. Moreover, other studies have shown additional reductions in the nutrient content of magnesium, calcium, copper, iron, phosphate, potassium and polyphenols, along with increases in heavy metals, insecticides and herbicides.[11] Adding insult to injury, the carcinogens Perfluorooctanoic acid and perfluorooctane sulfonate (PFOS), also known as forever chemicals because they latch on within your body, never to leave, are in high concentrations in many watering sources used for these fruits and vegetables.[12,13]

At the Champ residence we have planted and lovingly maintain a large backyard garden. This garden provides my family with a steady supply of tasty and nutritious organic vegetables, grown from homemade fertilizer and (hopefully) polyfluoroalkyl-free water. Of course, the climate in Pittsburgh does limit our year-round ability to grow and consume these vegetables. Store-bought vegetables are nearly always mono-cropped and grown in an environment with inadequate soil nutrition, thus these vegetables can be reasonably expected to be suboptimal and ever-declining in nutrition yield as well. My family and I eat plenty of vegetables and nutrient-dense animal-based foods like aged raw cheese, pastured eggs, grass-fed beef, wild boar, salmon, cod, shrimp, squid and octopus, but some of these animals are often eating plants that are grown in depleted soil as well. Thus, the curse of low-nutrient soils is a levied tax that gains compound interest throughout the food chain and through multiple generations.

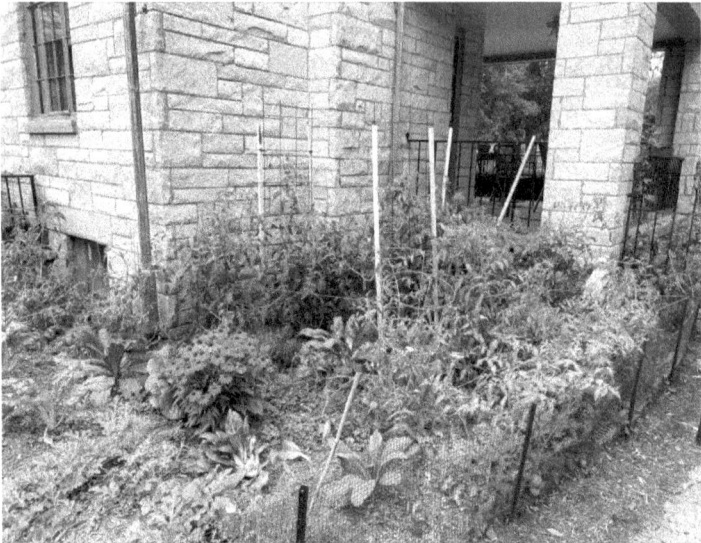

The Champ family garden is generally overrun with tomatoes from seeds brought over from Italy in the 1800s. The garden uses compost from a bin in the back corner of the yard and utilizes PFAS-free water.

The quality of our nutrition is absolutely vital, as our body critically relies on their micronutrients to properly function, repair DNA and cellular damage, and ultimately fight diseases like cancer. Some cancer research experts like Bruce Ames have hypothesized that this deficiency may be a major precursor to cancer, as it leaves our cells with an inability to repair DNA damage.[14] Ames is no slouch when it comes to cancer, as the test that holds his namesake—the Ames Test—is the standard for quickly assessing whether substances and chemicals cause DNA mutations and are carcinogenic (i.e. cause cancer). His work has also has linked the consumption of 30 vitamins and minerals with healthy aging.[15] Newer data have strengthened Ames' hypotheses, revealing links with several cancer diagnoses and vitamin and mineral deficiency.[16]

As a result, for many of us it is prudent to supplement when necessary. As for me, I engage in the following regimen:

1. Vitamin D3: I weigh just shy of 200lb and take the equivalent of 2,000 IU per day. In the spring, summer and early fall I get my vitamin D through the sun only. Otherwise, I always attempt to get vitamin D from my food year-round, including full-fat dairy (e.g. butter, cream and cheese), fatty fish and whole eggs.

2. Vitamin K2: I take 45 mcg daily, though I prefer to get as much K2 from food as possible. Optimal foods include fermented cheese, fermented vegetables (kraut and kimchi), egg yolks, grass-fed butter, ground beef (ideally with organ meat included), fatty meats and heavy cream in my morning coffee.

3. Fish Oil: I take 3 grams daily in the morning. While I aim to get as much Omega-3 as possible through my diet by eating fatty fish, oysters when available, grass-fed beef, egg yolks from pastured chickens, and full fat dairy from grass-fed cows, due to shortcuts

producing our crops and livestock, these levels are not always where they should be. Please note that Omega-3s in nuts and plant sources contain a different type of Omega-3, in the form of ALA (Alpha lipoic acid), and only a small amount of this type is converted to active forms in our body. On the other hand, EPA (Eicosapentaenoic acid) and DHA (Docosahexaenoic acid) are found in certain fish and animal foods from appropriately raised and fed animals that freely roam the pasture, eating their appropriate diet of bugs for chickens and grass for cows. For example, Omega-3 is found in significantly higher levels in the fat of cows that are fed 100% grass diets.[15] The same can be said for vitamin E, beta-carotene and several other nutrients and vitamins.

4. Magnesium: I take this at night, and usually in the form of several available types like malate, citrate and glycinate. I take the equivalent of 150-300mg per day several hours before the *Golden Girls* reruns come on. Again, I try to get most of my magnesium through real foods, although due to poor local soil management and mono-cropping such foods are generally low in magnesium. Candidate magnesium-

rich foods include almonds, full-fat dairy from grass-fed cows, leafy greens, broccoli, okra, blackberries, dark chocolate (look up the type to assess for lead and cadmium levels), avocados, and fatty fish, as well as assorted herbs and spices. I will also eat high-magnesium bananas after a workout if I am trying to gain weight.

5. Turmeric: I take a curcumin extract with piperine; piperine enhances curcumin absorption. It is a mixture that ends up being around 2,000mg. We also cook with turmeric, but admittedly do not have enough recipes in our rotation that call for it. This is a supplement you want to run by your physician if you plan on adding it to your regimen as it can interact with some medical treatments.

I hope that as you read through my supplements list you contemplated our discussions across the previous chapters. Most of the foods that provide the vitamins above—particularly K2, D3, magnesium, and fatty acids—are vilified by mainstream nutritionists, primarily on account of their fat content. Ponder that as you strive to ensure your foods are as "high-quality" as possible, i.e. containing the highest available amount of vitamins and nutrients.

This list is by no means exhaustive, and once more I will emphasize that I try to limit my vitamins via supplements and maximize absorbing my nutrients and minerals via food. For instance, I use high mineral salt daily—often mixing it with water and drinking it—-as it contains a full spectrum of health-boosting minerals. Salt is yet another ally painted as a "bad guy" by dietary recommendations handed down from the nutrition world's ivory tower establishment of yesteryear, and upon closer inspection does not make sense to restrict if you are healthy and exercise. In other words, if you are still following a low-salt diet recommendation, please STOP as there is no solid data to support such adverse claims; in fact, if you eat a healthy diet and exercise, you are likely not getting enough salt by default due to salt loss by perspiration. A famous study on salt intake conducted by Andrew Mente known as the PURE study assessed over 133,000 individuals and found that a low salt diet in individuals without hypertension was associated with a *higher* risk of cardiovascular disease.[17] Be it salt, supplements or soil-grown produce, it's well past time to take a wrecking ball to the ivory tower.

11

WE ARE NOT ALCHEMISTS: POOR RESULTS AND SICKNESS FOLLOW POOR BEHAVIORS

"I fell off the wagon for a month."

"The kids were home from school."

"It was the holidays."

"My spouse keeps buying junk food."

"It's summer and I like to have drinks at the pool."

"I keep getting sick."

"I don't understand why I am not achieving my goals."

I often hear this last sentence from Nutrition Sessions clients who just don't seem to be improving rapidly enough on their health journeys. And when they do not see the needle moving with fat loss, they find excuses or justifications, typically in the form of one of the first six comments or something similar. Conducting a deeper dive with more probing questions often reveals even more of the usual suspects: lots of TV, lots of "digital cigarettes" (i.e. screens and devices) usage, inadequate sleep, inadequate mobility and inadequate nutrients and vitamins.

Let's recap the laundry list of the basics we've established in this book:

1. Eating for vitamins and nutrients

2. Moving often/constantly throughout the day, every day

3. Getting adequate sleep (8 hours)

4. Interspersing intense activity/lifting heavy weights

5. Stimulating your brain and letting it rest

If we can't even check the above five boxes, perhaps we should be modifying that last sentence:

"No wonder I can never achieve my goals."

Far too often we express surprise or frustration when we are not improving or achieving our goals fast enough. Perhaps a prudent first step is to change our point of view to one that incorporates a healthy dose of reality. We cannot magically maximize our situation if we are going against our body's innate requirements for cellular function, repair and regeneration. We cannot expect magic, nor can we expect our bodies to be alchemists that turn lead to gold: if we put garbage in, we cannot expect gold but rather garbage out. Poor results and sickness follow poor behaviors.

For instance, the meat of grass-fed cows contains significantly more Omega-3 fatty acids, conjugated linoleic acid (CLA) and other essential vitamins and nutrients when compared to the meat of corn-fed cows. Grass is the natural diet of cows, as their multiple stomachs ferment it and then they digest the bacteria. Like us, cows are not alchemists. They cannot turn an unnatural diet that their bodies are unable to process into nutritional gold, and then they get both sick and fat. The result is less healthy meat and an increase in bovine infections requiring antibiotics. Poor results and sickness follow poor behaviors.

We cannot do one thing and expect another, regardless of whether the kids are home, it is the holidays or there is a *Golden Girls* marathon on the tube all week. If we do not fuel our body with high octane, rev the engine to max cycles periodically, and then rest and recharge daily, then we cannot expect it to magically function at its fullest. And we certainly cannot expect it to avoid breaking down.

In my prior books, I wrote at length about the importance of self-care using the poetic words of the French philosopher Voltaire:

Il faut cultiver son jardin." (In English: "Let us cultivate our garden.")

If a patch of soil we are responsible for tending is not nurtured and cultivated it will quickly become overrun with weeds, unwelcome intruders which will crowd out and choke the healthy, nutritious plants and beautiful flowers. Thinking that vegetables and flowers can magically grow in such a cluttered environment is a ridiculous premise. So then, why is it not equally ridiculous to believe our own bodies will produce the fruits we desire without the proper till and toil to keep the weeds away?

Poor results and sickness follow poor behaviors. We are not alchemists; our bodies and minds require adequate nutrition, stimulation, rest, repair and regeneration. If we are not even providing the bare necessities, perhaps it is time to stop being so shocked with the results (or lack thereof).

Reversing Our Thought Process

Oftentimes, I hear clients question why they are unhealthy or why they just can't drop that weight. It is time to reverse that thought process. If we are not following the above laundry list, we should be examining why we aren't achieving our health goals. For instance, when creating a client workout regimen at the EOC we consider all the factors that could stand in the way of recovery: lack of sleep, stress, medication (chemotherapy or targeted agents), and hormonal changes (anti-estrogen, testosterone blocking medications, or menopause). If none of the factors—or better yet, let's call them "anti-factors" since they are directly working against our recovery—are present, the workout can be intense or high-volume. However, for each one of the anti-factors present, we have to ratchet down the intensity to ensure adequate recovery and reduce the risk of injury to our client. Obviously, we cannot expect optimal results when such anti-factors are blockers to maximum physical performance and efficiency.

We must approach our health the same way. How many anti-factors are present? Or, to strike a chord closer to the truth, how many of these are self-induced? For each one, we can expect a lower chance of reaching our health goals. Some of the anti-factors may lead to other compounding anti-factors. For instance, if we stay up late on devices at night we may not achieve adequate sleep, accelerating our trajectory towards derailing our health goals. In the same vein, staying up late may precipitate waking up late and not starting the day with adequate nutrition for breakfast or meal preparation for lunch, and now one anti-factor has quickly morphed into three, and we are getting not linearly but exponentially further away from achieving optimal health.

None of us—save a handful of enterprising rare-earth metal scientists out there— are alchemists. But you don't have to have a metallurgy PhD or the recipe for gold bars to understand the principle that the purer the ingredients put into a mix, the purer the resulting substance. From chemists to chefs to car mechanics to artists, this principle is roundly applied: we want to minimize the impurities—i.e., anti-factors—to achieve the finest final product. We must treat ourselves, our bodies and our health no differently. Anti-factors are those things that constantly work against us. Televisions and devices are anti-factors for sleep and adequate nutrition, not to mention mental health and avoiding anxiety and impulsive and addictive behaviors. Packaged foods are anti-factors for nutrition, as they promote overeating and convenience, while encouraging a pathologic relationship with food.

The good news is that those same anti-factors that keep us from recovering after a workout are the same culprits that elevate our anxiety and depression levels, bring about ailments and illnesses, and generally derail our winding journey to general health and wellness. By acknowledging, addressing and improving on these, we can kill more than a dozen birds with one stone.

Excuses and justifications come and go. Do you care enough to make it happen?

12

FINAL WORDS

I am operating in an industry where many of my peers seem to be fine with seeing clients remain overweight for the majority of their working lives and continuing to give them ineffective advice. In this world it can be difficult to go against the grain, and in doing so I have discovered that many dietitians that I have never met dislike me. Some even hate me. Moreover, I have discovered that it's not just me: I have colleagues around the country that are quite successful at helping individuals lose fat, gain muscle, and look and feel better... and they are also hated by masses of so-called "expert" researchers, nutritionists, dietitians and exercise gurus.

You would think that simply trying to get people to a healthier place is a noble occupation, and that any individuals who dedicate their lives to this task would be praised for their efforts. Unfortunately, it simply does not work like that, particularly in academia. People spend lots of time and money to learn nutritional recommendations from the 1970s and they do not want to hear that it was a waste or that they are required to move on from those views. A lack of the ability to critically think can further handcuff these individuals when it comes to self-assessment. Additionally, if a scientific body of work—newer research, or simply nutrition and exercise study results—further reveals that these views are an unfortunate relic of a misguided nutritional movement, their guardians quickly show their fangs as they kick and scream to protect their views, even if they are likely aware that the success rate of these views is close to zero. My friends and colleagues often ask how someone is able to give the same recommendations over and over again while watching those on the receiving end fail, and the answer is an incredible amount of stubbornness mixed with an unwillingness to approach any amount of critical thinking.

My mentor once told me, somewhat tongue-in-cheek, that after four years of BS he received a BS in Dietetics. It takes critical thinkers to critically think about what they are learning and what they have learned. It takes an even more complex thought process to avoid becoming too attached to what has been learned and come to the realization that it is healthy to question our professions. If we in this industry deeply want to help people improve their health and reach their goals, that desire should be the driving force. And if we are striking out at this task 95% of the time, perhaps it is time to reconsider our approach.

The disdain I experience coming from my peers is worth it at the end of the day, because the feeling of accomplishment and fulfillment I get from witnessing my breakthrough clients living their best lives and looking and feeling their best due to their efforts is all the reward that is needed. The envious egos can be angry, but they are nothing but angry bystanders—antiquated dinosaurs of academia and medicine that are getting passed by, nothing but a blur in the periphery soon to be in the past and forgotten forever.

EPILOGUE:

FINITE GAMES AND YOUR HEALTH

In 1986 James Carse, Professor Emeritus of history and literature of religion at New York University, published a masterpiece of literature titled Finite and Infinite Games. In this very short but sweet book, Carse told us that:

"There are at least two kinds of games. One could be called finite, the other infinite. A finite game is played for the purpose of winning, an infinite game for the purpose of continuing the play."

Carse's book quickly became one of my favorites and remains at the top of my recommended list. I lend it out frequently, and this is likely why my copy is spewing at the seams with a worn cover and dozens of stained pages. Finite and Infinite Games does an incredible job at simplifying the major components of life into two black and white categories. Life, as Carse symbolically reminds us, cannot easily be separated into two, and the goal is rather to avoid the finite bounded games and instead focus on the infinite major one. Flying in the face of what we are consistently told by society and the media, the real goal of life is to engage in those long-term games where there are no victors. Forget the winners and losers, the goal is to simply be a player in the infinite game, which provides the ultimate goal in life: simply being part of it.

There are no gold star stickers in this game. No trophies or medals. No "pokes" or "likes" from someone we have not seen in 20 years on some social media app that monopolizes our time and makes us anxious and overstimulated in return. No comment posts from the guy we never liked in high school but are somehow now "friends" with on Twitter, rekindling a friendship that was never there to begin with. The infinite games could care less about these useless scoring metrics.

Health: The Infinite Game

During my initial read of Carse's masterpiece and every time I have returned to it, the analogies and parallels to a healthy lifestyle never fail to stand out. While most of the nutrition and health world—at least in the spotlight of the media—seems to fight over fad diets, calories, carbohydrates and eating or avoiding meat, consumerism continues to consume its victims, "Conveniencism" as I like to call it leaves us pining for and chasing the easiest and quickest, and the many facets of modern-day life actively promote a lifestyle composed of an infinite number of finite games that destroy our mental and physical health before our very own eyes.

These finite games are everywhere—right in front of our faces on billboards, ads, commercials, in our hospitals[9] and even in our schools. These activities do nothing to benefit our lives in truly meaningful ways, yet we continually push for more and more. We sit here fighting about what is the optimal diet while a majority of the population does not even consume real food and eats most meals in front of the TV or a device. Did your 30-Day Detox sell 30,000 copies? Congratulations, you won a finite game. Did your book actually leave people healthier and striving for more? Kudos, as then they have entered the infinite game with your help.

While the finite games seem rather easy to define, the infinite game, like the path to health, is a bit more cryptic. In Carse's words, "Infinite games are more mysterious—and ultimately more rewarding. They are unscripted and unpredictable; they are the source of true freedom." Talking heads may argue about the optimal path to health on social media, and achieving—or rather maintaining—health may be unglamorous, but this goal is a quintessential example of an infinite game we play.

Going Infinite for Your Health

We are all consumed by a series of finite games, and when it comes to our health these kinds of finite jousts are often a recipe for disaster. Advising people to exercise more and count calories while simultaneously inundating them with an unstoppable barrage of nudges that pushes them ever closer to falling down that slippery slope is a finite game that most will lose.

Yet Carse's seminal work—surely neither a health treatise nor a fad diet book—may have provided us an antidote to the madness, via an approach you will not see in many health books. Fad diet books continue to pop up left and right (finite games), and products and "hacks" are produced at an alarming rate and aggressively promoted as magic solutions to turn around our health (more finite games). Yet, the vast majority of us will never achieve optimal health until we turn a blind eye to finite games and instead focus on merely continuing to play the infinite game of life.

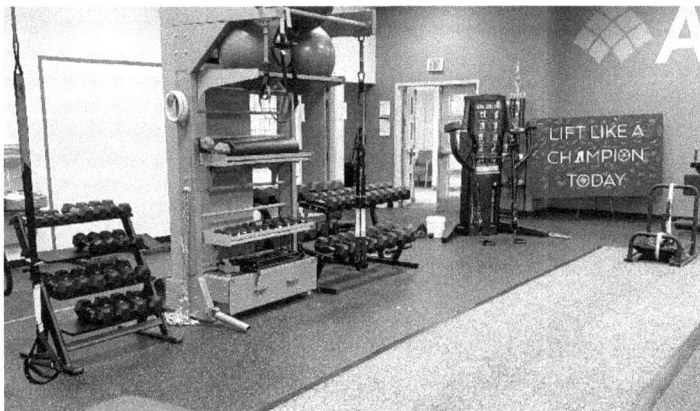

Above is the EOC, where the structured yet endless combinations and permutations of strength and conditioning, mobility, range of motion, targeting muscle groups from every angle exercises so as to never reach a plateau. The infinite game of resistance training is played so we can remain strong, mobile, and healthy throughout our lives and keep playing.

In Carse's own words: "a finite player seeks power… an infinite (player) displays self-sufficient strength. Finite games are theatrical, necessitating an audience… infinite ones are dramatic, involving participants." What greater self-sufficient strength is there than fortifying our own health? Our health requires no audience, just willing participants—-at the end of the day, it is just us facing ourselves in the mirror.

Sounds simple enough, but rest assured the allure of finite games constantly calls to us, subliminally beckoning while threatening our infinite game of health. For instance, in today's American society we are surrounded with constant temptations that constitute finite games at their worst:

1. Winning by obtaining the cheapest products available (a time sink that promotes focusing on quantity over quality, a disaster when it comes to food specifically)

2. Grouping the entire world into two finite political classes, demonizing one or the other, and watching news shows programmed to make us angry, divided, and, much like processed foods, addicted

3. Attempting to win at finite dietary strategies and gimmicky exercise routines instead of focusing on a

general health and proactive lifestyle that respects oneself and others

4. Attempting to win the ultimate finite game, social media, by pining for addictive "likes" and acknowledgment from people of little meaning or consequence (many of whom you've never even met in real life), leading you to post toxic comments and denigrating pictures of yourself that you would have never imagined even a few years ago

There are no winners in this finite game, only losers. You can ignore these finite games and instead turn towards the infinite games:

1. A trip to the gym is a finite game; a mixed and varied exercise regimen incorporated within your lifestyle is the ultimate infinite game. For those involved, there are no infinite winners and losers, only those who keep playing. For those who quit, their health loses and they lose.

2. A healthy home: There are no medals, thumbs up or "likes" for cleaning your house, doing the dishes or helping your spouse cook meals. Yet, these activities will promote a healthy and happy marriage and leave you continuing to play that infinite game.

3. Hunting and gathering high quality food, cooking with family and friends and then gathering around the dinner

table to enjoy the nutritious food is an ultimate infinite game. It is an activity that constitutes the basic essence of being human, a timeless and eternal act that spiritually connects us with every member of our species past, present, and future. There are no prizes and short-term goals, no medals and no fodder for egos. This infinite game provides long-term health, better relationships with friends and families, and an appreciation for life that may take decades to realize. There are no short-term winners and losers.

4. Living your life to the fullest, working hard, optimizing arete (the pursuit of human excellence), and always fare bella figura (doing well and behaving good) rarely provide short-term victories, but in the infinite game of life you will always come out on top.

Don't have enough time to do this? How much time do you spend watching television (Golden Girls excluded, of course!) and browsing social media outlets? Remove these and ask yourself if you still do not have enough time. Carse has an answer to this as well: "The infinite player in us does not consume time but generates it. Because infinite play is dramatic and has no scripted conclusion, its time is time lived and not time viewed."

Finite games are played for the purpose of winning. Infinite games are played for the purpose of merely playing. The former is the epitome of short-term reward; the latter is a never-ending process of finding deeper meaning and deeper purpose that leads to overall deeper satisfaction in life. Pursuing and maintaining personal health is not a short-term chase, it is an epic lifelong odyssey we are required to keep on playing from our moment of self-awareness to our moment of death. A physically and mentally healthy lifestyle is the ultimate infinite game. If you haven't been playing the right way, it's never too late to change your strategy.

References

1.   Hess, J. M. et al. Dietary Guidelines Meet NOVA: Developing a Menu for A Healthy Dietary Pattern Using Ultra-Processed Foods. J. Nutr. 153, 2472–2481 (2023).

2.   Phinney, S. D., LaGrange, B. M., O'Connell, M. & Danforth Jr, E. Effects of aerobic exercise on energy expenditure and nitrogen balance during very low calorie dieting. Metabolism 37, 758–765 (1988).

3.   Van Cauter, E., Polonsky, K. S. & Scheen, A. J. Roles of Circadian Rhythmicity and Sleep in Human Glucose Regulation. Endocr. Rev. 18, 716–738 (1997).

4.   Caan, B. J. et al. Association of Muscle and Adiposity Measured by Computed Tomography With Survival in Patients With Nonmetastatic Breast Cancer. JAMA Oncol. 4, 798 (2018).

5.   Kurita, Y. et al. Sarcopenia is a reliable prognostic factor in patients with advanced pancreatic cancer receiving FOLFIRINOX chemotherapy. Pancreatology 19, 127–135 (2019).

6.   Phillips, S. M., Chevalier, S. & Leidy, H. J. Protein 'requirements' beyond the RDA: implications for optimizing health. Appl. Physiol. Nutr. Metab. 41, 565–572 (2016).

7.   Trommelen, J. et al. The anabolic response to protein ingestion during recovery from exercise has no upper limit in magnitude and duration in vivo in humans. Cell Reports Med. 4, (2023).

8.   Yanovski, J. A. et al. A prospective study of holiday weight gain. N. Engl. J. Med. 342, 861–7 (2000).

9.   Champ, C. E., Iarrobino, N. A. & Haskins, C. P. Hospitals Lead by Poor Example: An Assessment of Snacks, Soda, and Junk Food Availability in Veterans Affairs Hospitals. Nutrition 0, (2018).

10.   Davis, D. R., Epp, M. D., Riordan, H. D. & Davis, D. R. Changes in USDA food composition data for 43 garden crops, 1950 to 1999. J. Am. Coll. Nutr. 23, 669–682 (2004).

11.   Hasanaliyeva, G. et al. Effects of Agricultural Intensification on Mediterranean Diets: A Narrative Review. Foods 2023, Vol. 12, Page 3779 12, 3779 (2023).

12.   Li, Y. et al. Review on plant uptake of PFOS and PFOA for environmental cleanup: potential and implications. Environ. Sci. Pollut. Res. 28, 30459–30470 (2021).

13.   Lal, M. S., Megharaj, M., Naidu, R. & Bahar, M. M. Uptake of perfluorooctane sulfonate (PFOS) by common home-grown vegetable plants and potential risks to human health. Environ. Technol. Innov. 19, 100863 (2020).

14.   Ames, B. N. DNA damage from micronutrient deficiencies is likely to be a major cause of cancer. Mutat. Res. - Fundam. Mol. Mech. Mutagen. 475, 7–20 (2001).

15.   Smith, C. J. et al. Bruce Nathan Ames - Paradigm shifts inside the cancer research revolution. Mutat. Res. Rev. Mutat. Res. 787, (2021).

16.   Venturelli, S., Leischner, C., Helling, T., Burkard, M. & Marongiu, L. Vitamins as Possible Cancer Biomarkers: Significance and Limitations. Nutrients 13, (2021).

17.   Mente, A. et al. Associations of urinary sodium excretion with cardiovascular events in individuals with and

without hypertension: a pooled analysis of data from four studies. Lancet 388, 465–475 (2016).

INDEX

Other Work by the Author:

MISGUIDED
MEDICINE

SECOND EDITION

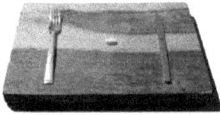

The Truth Behind Ill-Advised Medical Recommendations
and How to Take Health Back into Your Hands

Colin E. Champ, M.D.

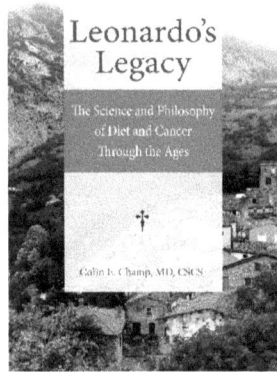

Leonardo's
Legacy

The Science and Philosophy
of Diet and Cancer
Through the Ages

Colin E. Champ, MD, CSCS

www.ingramcontent.com/pod-product-compliance
Lightning Source LLC
Chambersburg PA
CBHW060500280326
41933CB00014B/2802